THE THIRD YEAR

--An Africa-American medical student's odyssey through hope, death, and redemption

by

George L. Saunders, III, MD

Paperback ISBN: 978-1-7330603-0-1

Ebook ISBN: 978-1-7330603-2-5

DEDICATION

to my mother, Hazel,

who gave me the strength to master and growbeyond it,

to "Tim" who suffered and

succumbed to its pain,

to All those who,withcourage,would brave

the Third Year

this work is dedicated.

--G.L.S.

ACKNOWLEDGMENTS

There are many who helped me in the creation of this book. Here are but a few--My mother, Hazel and my sister, Amanda, guided me to medical school and a better life.

The rest of my family, including father, George, my other mothers, Frances and Dorene, my wife Marietta, daughters Nzingha, Makare, and Keyanna, brothers, sisters, nieces, nephews, cousins, aunts, uncles.

Richard Butcher, MD, mentor and consummate Family Physician, Nolan Penn, PhD, "priest-confessor," the Faculty of University of California at San Diego, School of Medicine, Jean and Harry Joynes, Bruce Patton and the Patton clan, my "son" Dr. James Fulwood.

Thank you all for sharing your love, knowledge, and your time

George L. Saunders, III, MD

Table of Contents

THE THIRD YEAR

THE THIRD YEAR

THE THIRD YEAR

THE THIRD YEAR

FORWARD

The time frame of The Third Year was 1977 to 1979. It was the eclipse of the Golden age of Medicine. Physicians had been the unquestioned masters of hospitals and clinics. Patients could be admitted simply for exhaustion with no question asked. The advent of the CAT scan precluded many unnecessary surgeries and the Ultrasound was a new and largely untried modality. Health care was changing to highly accurate and expensive, science-dominated procedures with the loss of the personal practice of Medicine.

CHAPTER 1

I am a poet-warrior caught in the fray of a battlefield as pervasive, boundless, and intangible as the human spirit. The battle is real, tangible. I taste its reality with my every breath. I am enveloped by it, chained and enslaved by it. At times, it exalts me to never before dreamed heights. I love this battlefield. I hate it. It is my mother, my lover, my friend. It is the confidante of my deepest fears and betrayer of my most fragile secrets. It is my greatest challenge, and contains what truth and beauty I know.

--Writings of the Poet-Priest

I**n truth, the** third year was not the third year at all for it came after I was forced to take pathology and the second year 0f medical school yet again.

The third year came after a year of intense searching, a year in which I gave myself over to the dedicated pursuit of knowledge of medicine and myself. The third year was not the third year for in my anxiousness to simply pass in the eyes of my evaluators, I had fallen in their eyes and, more importantly, my own. I tried with futile abandon to modify, lessen their pronouncement, but my efforts were as utter a failure as my academic performance.

I was doomed. For a long time afterward, I was a ghost unto myself, trying desperately to become one with myself again. Only a few weeks before, my marriage to the beautiful Grace had gone from worried silences to widening separation. Thus, the edict of the priests under whose tutelage I remained, was only the second greatest failure of my entire life.

In the year that preceded that which I call the third year, I determined that not pride, humiliation, nor anger would stop me from learning all that I possibly could. I determined that I would grow because of the experience, not fall, that I would excel though it was easier to falter. I attacked pathology, the very essence of the basis of medicine with a ferocious vigor. At first, I studied with one eye always seeking the approval of the priests. But later as I performed well easily on the examinations, I vowed to study for me alone. It was then I realized that striving for excellence in my own eyes, would get me far beyond "passing" in anyone's eyes.

Learning became a joy. When I was not studying, I passed many sun-laden hours listening to the sound of my heartbeat, calling to white-bellied gulls and whispering my cherished secrets to the wind. I began to know myself again. I searched for inner peace and the love of my lost bride.

Thus, passed a year in which I founded my knowledge of medicine for many years to come and in which I renewed my search for self. It was at times painfully lonely and at times gentle and pleasant.

CHAPTER 2

Grant us patience in the face of adversity and new priests.

--prayer for July of the nurses and attending priests of the House of the God of Life.

I **arrived** on the wards after two days of lectures. I arrived on the wards, hallowed halls of the God of Life, my white coat gleaming and my new, black bag smooth and unmarred, filled with instruments shining and unused. I stood with a group of three medical students who, like me, were to receive instruction by the priests of the God of Surgery. Fear showed clearly on our fresh-scrubbed faces as we were yet untried in this the final proving ground of the priests of the God of Life. It was here on the wards, that the great physician I knew myself to be would either excel or fail utterly. There was no middle ground. The challenge lay before me. I shook only slightly. I glanced at the student-priests at my side and smiled nervously. I was not alone, in my trepidation. "Where's Dr. Raymond?" one of the bolder of our group ventured to a tall green-suited woman. She eyed us disdainfully, marking closely our tooth paste-fresh smiles and the many-creased greens we had donned. "He's in room two." She pointed to a thick wooden door with a small window, then passed swiftly down the hallway, disappearing behind a second closed door.

We stood before the indicated door, peering through the small window. A large spotlight focused on the open abdomen of a man whose face I could not see.

"Can we go in?"

"Maybe we should wait."

A few seconds passed.

"They might be there for a long time."

"I want to see."

We pushed into the operating room, terrified that our very presence would somehow abolish the sterility of the operating field. A few eyes left the patient's red abdomen, inquiring of us.

"You the new medical students?" a voice behind a mask asked. "Yes."

"Yes." we answered in staccato chorus.

"Are you Dr. Raymond?" one of the medical students asked. Raymond was the name of the chief resident of surgery.

"No, I'm Bob Raymond." A serious young priest looked up briefly.

"Are we supposed to scrub?" one of the student-priests asked.

"No, just watch." Raymond answered. The student-priest was crushed. "You can come closer."

We approached the operating field, leaving the far wall for only the first time since we had entered the operating room. The assisting nurse, before whom a multitude of instruments was arrayed, eyed us suspiciously. We moved toward the far end of the table. Raymond introduced the other resident and interns of his team. Each priest nodded as his name was called. Each name I quickly forgot, and each face blended into a sea of green masks. The surgery we watched was a very difficult one for both the patient and operators. Later, I was to find that the abdominal-perineal resection, or A-P resection, entailed the removal of the rectum and anus en bloc and bringing out the remaining end of bowel in a colostomy. It was done for rectal cancer and had a long list of possible complications. From my vantage point, I could see the face of this man who appeared in his forties. I studied the brown, almost red, handle bar mustache, the shaven head. The man was imbued with the stillness, silence, and pallor of death. His respirations kept the slow cadence of a funeral dirge. It seemed that a such a face as this could never drink of the waters of life again.

My attention returned to the operating field. The chief resident diligently instructed one of the junior residents in the technique of the procedure. This was a great kindness as cases like this one were rare and belonged indisputably to the chief resident.

Two of the priests broke away from their colleagues to begin work on the rectum. They used uneven, almost hacking strokes. I was surprised that the precision I had always envisioned as the hallmark of the priests of the God of the Blade was nowhere evinced.

□ □ □ □

As a rubber tube was placed where his rectum had been and a puff of pink intestine protruded from the man's belly, I witnessed my first miracle in the House of the God of Life. The anesthesiologist adjusted several knobs and valves, then the patient who had seemed inexorably in the jaws of Death awakened. More than this he moved of his own volition. Still, I thought, it can only be a short time before he loses the final match with Death.

The students gathered uncertainly at the sink. "What was that operation?" Bob Dausman asked. He was balding and combed a few strands over the top of his head in a half-hearted effort to conceal a bare spot.

"I don't know." Mark Polsky answered. Mark, an unquestioned scholar, had a way of making whatever he said sound super intelligent.

I shrugged my shoulder.

"Do we all go with them?" Bob asked.

"They're going to split us up." Gail Reed answered.

"Until they split us up, I guess we'd better follow them."

The three male student-priests followed the surgeons into the locker room. Gail went to the nurse's locker room to change as it was the only place in the operating room suite where women could change. We all met again, resident-priests in long white coats, interns and students in short lab jackets, as afternoon rounds began.

□ □ □ □

The next morning, at 6:30 A.M., we again reported for rounds, but with a considerably less romanticized vision of the wards brought on acutely by the ungodly hour and the foreshortening of sleep which it entailed. We passed through the section of 5-North where the E-service patients were bedded.

"Good morning. How are you, Mr. Mondini?" The assistant resident asked.

"I'm O.K., doc." He managed a little smile. I looked at the face of the man who had just the day before undergone an A-P resection. Amazement purged the last remnants of sleep from my head. This man whom I had been certain would be carried away in the jaws Of Death, sat before me looking as if he might be recovering from a cold but nothing more serious.

"You have any pain?"

"Just a little."

"That's to be expected," the resident answered.

"Any fever?" Raymond, the chief resident, asked the intern.

"No. No fever."

"Let's look at the wound." We stood around the patient while the intern gathered items for a dressing change. The wound looked good. The priests of the God of the Blade were pleased. The team moved on. I stayed back, taking a last look at the man who had seemed so recently beyond the domain of the God of Life. There were many mysteries of the priesthood I needed to learn. This man and his surgery were but one.

CHAPTER 3

Ritual serves many functions. It, at once, teaches, re-enforces, needed information and affirms our service to Life and the many Gods that serve the God of Life. Perhaps as important, it unifies the priesthood as a single order, whose mission is the preservation of life and the alleviation of suffering.

--Lectures of the Academy
of Priests of the God of Life

W**e watched** silently as the priests performed their ablations, offering brown foam to the demi-god, Cleanliness. They were clad in the green hoods and robes of the priests of the Cutting Sect. They prayed to their God, the God of the Knife, that their dance of distraction might allow them to steal yet a few beads of time for the man on whom they would operate. They prayed to the God of Life and the God of the Blade for sure hands and sharp ears that they might avoid the paths of Infection and Hemorrhage, obedient and ever-watchful servants of the God of Death. We watched as each priest scrubbed his arms to the elbow, then rinsed under the holy water. As the priests shook the remnants of the holy liquid from their bodies, each paused at the sink. Each looked deeply into the pattern of splashing water as if reading signs there as ancient priests had once read entrails. One by one, the highest followed by the lowest, the priests left the glistening bowl to enter the land where Death stalked and was followed closely by grim and merciless attendants. After the lowest of the priests had entered, we, the medical students, the untouchables of the priesthood, passed through the wooden doors to stand as silent spectators on an arduous journey.

CHAPTER 4

The power of the priesthood is inexplicable and wondrous.

--lectures, Academy of the Priests of the God of Life

T**he green tiled** corridors were at their usual moderate morning pace. As I traveled the main hallway to 5-North, I turned down the passageway leading to B-pod. A small rectangular slip of paper lay on the counter top. I read the addressograph stamp.

Sally entered the nurse's station. I liked Sally. I liked her a lot. She was warm, attractive, knowledgeable. She had gone out of her way to teach me how to draw blood on difficult patients. So that I might gain more skill, she had agreed to call me when there was blood to draw.

"Mr. Kinney needs to have blood drawn." She looked at me with brown eyes that would make stone melt. "I tried, but I couldn't get it." She said this evenly, without mockery, though two weeks before it had been she who had taught the young student-priest how to draw blood.

"I'll give it my best shot." I answered as I headed for the clean utility room.

"Oh, I know you can do it." She called to me. I smiled. There was a noisy clatter, as I searched for the first two of my favorite weapons in the minor skirmishes of blood and gore. My fingers fell upon the familiar black cover of a 22-gauge needle which I placed upon a ten-cc syringe. As I entered the patient's room, I donned my final, and most powerful, tool--a face, grim as that of Death itself.

"Hello, Mr. Kinney. I'm here to draw your blood." I pushed up my sleeve.

"Hi, doc." A pale thin, half-shaven man looked up at me from a rumpled maze of white sheets. "I'm glad you're here."

He wore a blue hospital gown. Mr. Kinney spoke rapidly when excited. He spoke quickly as I stood before him. "Those nurses are O.K., doc, but they can't draw blood on me. I got no veins. You see?" He extended pale vessel-less arms toward me. "I wouldn't let her try on me again after she missed the first time." He continued, barely pausing for a breath. "The guys who come around in the morning couldn't get it either. I'm not trying to cause no trouble, doc." He looked at me imploringly. "I just thought it would be better to have the doctor draw the blood."

"Hm-m-m." How am I going to get this blood? I thought. I said, "This is going to be tight." I knotted the rubber tourniquet.

"That's O.K."

The blood drawing ritual began. It was always the same. I tied the tourniquet on first one arm, then the other. I spent up to fifteen minutes looking for a suitable vein. I always felt extreme sympathy for the patient as I watched the same expression of pained anguish and tolerance as I pushed the needle into the arm. I was always relieved and surprised (though I almost never missed even in the beginning of the third year) when the precious liquid appeared in the tube.

"That's it." I told Mr. Kinney as I gathered my tools.

"Thanks, doc." He spoke with more relief than gratitude.

"You're welcome." I carried the still warm liquid to the nurse's station. Sally looked up as I approached.

"Got some blood?"

"Yes, here it is."

"Here," she extended her hand, "I'll take that for you." I handed her the tubes. I watched Sally as she placed the tubes with the lab slips. She had fully expected me to get the blood though she had taught me the technique. The patient had fully expected that I would get the blood. I had gotten the blood. As I turned to leave, I was less impressed with the skill of one priest-cadet than with the power and awe given by so many to those who wore the robes of the priesthood.

CHAPTER 5

Each new situation is marked by at least one moment of crisis. Growth is the process of mastering these crises.

--an unknown philosopher

E**nter Joel Baker,** my first chief resident. Enter a figure bigger than life itself. Raymond lasted but a day before he left the E service where I had been assigned. His replacement, Joel, was an often condescending and distant mass of flesh who stood a few inches less than six feet but managed to tower over the tallest of the priests of the E service.

Joel was to be feared. Everyone knew this, the assistant resident, the interns. The medical students knew this also by some process akin to telepathy. He carried power as a huge club which he seldom used blatantly as the threat was far more effective. More than these, I found Joel to be fair. He expected no more out of his house staff than he was willing to do himself. Moreover, as he once told me, the medical students and interns, were expected to know only a few patients as any time, while he had to know all the patients on a service which sometimes rose to over thirty.

For reasons which are unknown, Joel liked me. After I got to know the priest under whose tread the ground seemed to tremble, he spent many hours teaching me the arts of surgery. This I saw him do with only one other person during the time I remained under his tutelage.

One of my classmates spoke to me over lunch. "Where are you at?"

"The V.A."

"Which service?"

"E service."

"D service?"

"No, *E* service."

"You're with Joel Baker."

"Yes", I answered. It always amazed me that while I had difficulty remembering the names of the doctors of my own team, other students as busy as I, knew the names and dispositions of all the interns and residents of each service. "Ugh." My colleague answered, thrusting out his jaw for emphasis.

"What do you mean?"

My interlocutor, a third-year medical student as myself, sucked the last of a carton of chocolate milk. The empty container made a sound like cracking pop-corn while his pursed lips tried to extract the last drop of liquid. "I heard Joel is hard to work with. He gives everybody a hard time. Fred Rocker said he was a real asshole. He said he couldn't stand him."

"He's O.K. to me." I answered, truthfully. "I get along with him fine."

"E is a busy service."

"Yeah." I agreed. "We get lots of cases."

□ □ □ □

"Joel find you?" Schom, one of the three interns on E service asked. It had been a busy morning. The entire team had been running since six-thirty.

"No." I answered. It was a little past one in the afternoon.

"He's looking for you."

"O.K., thanks."

The intern, Roger Speights, approached. He moved slowly, pushing an I.V. pole and stretcher before him. I went to help Roger.

"Where's he going?" I asked indicating the patient on the stretcher.

"B pod." I turned the head of the stretcher. A clear plastic tube protruded from the man's nose. His deeply yellow skin made a sharp contrast with the hospital white sheets. The man seemed acutely ill. The wrist band said Daniel Straight.

"You see Joel?" Roger asked.

"No."

"He wanted you for something." A moment later my name was called as I picked up the phone to page the chief resident.

"Yeah?" I answered.

"Joel's on the phone for you." I picked up the line Joel was on. Joel's voice was crisp. "There's a patient named Straight who's going to the O.R. in fifteen minutes. I want an H & P on the chart by the time he gets there."

I was dumb-founded. "O.K., Joel." I laid down the receiver. The time it took me to perform a complete history and physical and then write it up had diminished considerably while I was on surgery. If I hurried it took me only two and a half hours. Fifteen minutes?

"Did you go over the pre-op checklist for Straight?"
One of the nurses spoke behind me. I mumbled an answer. Fifteen minutes! I grabbed a history and physical sheet from the file cabinet. I galloped to the man's room.

"Mr. Straight", I told him my name. "I'm a third year medical
student. I'm going to examine you."

"Hi, doc."

"Mr. Straight, what brought you to the hospital?"

"I ain't been feeling too good for about three or four months. Today the pain got worse."

"Where's the pain at?"

"Here." He indicated a spot below his breastbone. I continued my questions, writing as he spoke. I obtained a review of systems as I examined the man who was soon to be given to the God of Surgery.

Twenty minutes after speaking with him on the phone, I saw Joel. Mr. Straight was on a stretcher just outside the operating room. As the double doors opened to admit our patient, I was writing the last of the history and physical.

"That H. & P. done?" Joel's tone was half-mocking, half-menacing.

I affixed my signature to the physical, then tossed the completed forms and clipboards onto the stretcher a half-second before the doors closed.

I straightened my harried frame, looked Joel directly in the eye and answered confidently, casually. "Yes." Joel looked at me briefly, amused. He turned to go to the locker room.

"Good." he tossed back over his shoulder.

"Thank you." I beamed.

CHAPTER 6

In the final analysis, though we serve our Gods, our Laws, we are human. We are neither completely unstained good nor irredeemable evil. We are creatures of flesh and blood, filled with aspirations and desires both base and noble We are called to a holy office, but as each human is holy, we are given no license with the title we cherish so highly. It is only our actions, guided by the purest of motives. which earn us the few privileges we deserve as priests. It is only as forgers of hope and givers of love that we are worthy of the respect that is given us.

--the Heretic-Priest

THE THIRD YEAR

Two A.M. On call. The intern who had hit the bed ten minutes after me was asleep. I looked at the ceiling, the snoring intern, and then at the ceiling. The tiredness was one deep in my bones, a dull aching. I was too tense to sleep. I dreaded having to get up again. I listened to the phone. I could hear it even when it did not ring. But it did ring. I hated that ringing. I cursed. It was after two A.M., closer to three and we had just gotten to bed. I was not required to get up. I could turn over, pretend I was asleep, or look at the intern listlessly as he dressed. That was what my colleagues did for the most part.

Most went to bed around twelve and could not be found until morning rounds. I shared the work of my intern usually until two o'clock, when they would not call me out of consideration for my tiredness (no greater than their own) or because they could go faster

alone. Often, I would not see them for hours at night. I knew the routine and initiated work on my own which I knew had to be done, only reporting to them once the work had been completed. For this, I earned their thanks and many a grateful, sleepy nod. The interns liked being on call with me because I was a work horse. They knew I could be depended upon to lighten their work load.

But the phone was ringing, really ringing, not just in my head the way it did when I startled awake only to hear the rattle of keys as the intern slipped off his pants. It was really ringing. I must have dosed off for my intern was gone. The phone stopped. I must have been dreaming. No, because there it goes again. I stumbled across the room in my underwear. Somebody stop the phone!!

"Hello-o-o!" I moaned.

"Hello, Dr. Dimino?" The voice was awake, crisp, polite.

"No, Dr. Dimino's not here."

"Do you know where he is?"

"He's on the floors somewhere. I don't know where."

"Oh, O.K." the voice at the other end said. I started to place the receiver back on the hook.

"Wait a minute." I called. "Hello?"

"Yes?" The woman's voice returned.

"I'm the medical student on surgery. Is it anything I can help you with?"

"Mr. Ramsey on 5-North has a temp of 102. Maybe you could . . . "

"I'll be down in a few minutes."

"O.K."

"By the way, how many days post-op is he?"

"He was operated on yesterday."

"O.K. I'll be down in a few minutes." I hung up the phone.

The cogs of my mind began to turn slowly. The process by which my brain functioned was one more akin to automatic recall rather than thinking. I had been through this too many times at the same ungodly hour to have to think. Besides, thinking required energy, a rare commodity at three A.M. Fever, first day after surgery. I slipped on my pants. Yes, yes, it was coming back to me. My feet sounded an empty patter as I left the almost cozy warmth of the on-call room. The most likely reason for the fever was atelectasis, a partial collapse of the lung caused by the patient not breathing deeply because of the pain of the surgery. I would have to check the patient first, of course, to rule out other less likely causes of fever. It was too early for a wound infection, but I would have to check, anyway.

A slightly rotund nurse in her mid-twenties looked up at me questioningly from behind a counter. She was disgustingly awake.

"Hello, you called about a patient?"

She looked at me as if I had just stepped off a spaceship. "We called you?"

"Yes, about a patient with a fever." Annoyance filled my voice.

"Are you sure it was us?"

"Yes. it was . . ." The familiarity of the settings edged into my consciousness. I was on 5-North, the ward where the E service patients were housed. The call had come from 5-East.

"Maybe it was another wing that called."

"I'm sorry, you're right." During the day, I would have attempted to take a short-cut to 5-East which required walking outside the building on a terrace, but in my half-asleep state I would certainly have gotten lost in the maze of staircases and passageways. I took the long route, instead, back to the central core and down the quarter mile of corridors to 5-East.

"Hi". I spoke to a nurse in her mid-thirties. She rose as I approached.

She held a chart in her hand. "Hi. Are you the medical student?"

"Yes." I told her my name.

"I'm Irene Hill. Here's Mr. Ramsey's chart. Would you like to take a look at it before you see the patient?" She handed me a metallic clipboard.

I thanked her as I took the chart. I scanned the pages of notes scribbled in illegible doctorese. I could make out that the patient had had some type of biliary tree surgery. Irene told me the exact nature of the surgery. He had had his gall bladder removed. She filled me in on his course as I searched for a medical student note, hoping to find at least one readable entry in the chart. No student had followed the patient. I was grateful for Irene's information.

□ □ □ □

I introduced myself to the patient. "How are you feeling? I asked the man.

"I guess, I'm doing O.K."

"They tell me you're running a fever."

"Yeah."

I went through the litany of questions that would help me localize any infection. He complained only of a mild cough. I removed my stethoscope, from my pants pocket. I probed, looked, and listened. There was nothing. I went to the clean utility room.

"What are you looking for?" Irene asked me.

"Blood culture bottles." I called. "I found them." I returned to the patient's room., I searched his arms for one good vein. There were none, only tiny blue flecks. Why do patients always have chicken veins at three in the morning? After obtaining the sample, I returned to the nurse's station and wrote the orders for blood, urine, and sputum. As I returned to the on-call room. My steps were made just the smallest bit lighter by a small sense of accomplishment. Dimino was still not in the room. The morning sun, rising as a fiery red ball in a sullen sky, found me sleeping and the intern's bed yet empty.

CHAPTER 7

There is in each of us that which is holy,
that which is Divine.
--The Heretic-Priest Speaks
to Laypeople

Close on the heels of the intern, I entered the room. Two nurses were at the old man's bedside. One spoke to him.

"Mr. Johnson, the doctor's here to examine you now."

"Hello, Mr. Johnson. I'm Dr. Dimino." It was an annoying habit of house staff when confronted by an uncooperative patient to shout, loudly, as if the volume of their voice alone was enough to vanquish all resistance.

Interestingly enough, I found that it usually worked.

Dimino waved the nurses away. "It's O.K. I'll take it from here." The older of the two nurses, a mildly obese woman with straw-colored hair, looked questioningly at the intern whose head of black hair rose only to her shoulder.

"I don't know," she said. Both nurses moved tentatively toward the door, then stopped.

"Mr. Johnson," the intern shouted, "I'm going to examine you now."

"Get away from me, you son of a bitch!" The old man hissed as he struck out at the intern. Both nurses rushed back to the patient. I stood a safe distance away, watching.

While the man continued to show belligerence toward the intern, I noted that he was gentle with the nurses.

"Mr. Johnson," the elder nurse scolded gently, "that's the doctor! He's here to examine you."

Dimino, who had been taken aback for a moment, proceeded once again, undaunted.

"O.K." For the second time, he waved the two nurses away. They did not move. "I have to examine you, Mr. Johnson." He placed his stethoscope on the man's chest. The old man was suddenly sitting up, coming toward the intern.

"God damn it!" he shouted vehemently. "I said don't touch me!"

"Mr. Johnson!" a nurse called.

"Mr. Johnson . . . " the intern shouted. His statement was cut short by a kick in the gut. The four struggled for a few seconds until Dimino was able to untangle himself from the Veteran.

"You O.K.?" one of the nurses asked the intern.

"Shit!" he shouted, his face scarlet. "Haldol five milligrams I.M. STAT!" He stormed out of the room. I followed, staying a few steps behind him to conceal my widening smile.

Mr. Johnson was only the third admission of the night. There
was a fourth patient whom neither the intern nor I had seen. He was a 43 year old with a positive oral cholecystogram, a positive history of nausea and vomiting, and abdominal pain. He was quite well as we spoke with him and was scheduled for the elective removal of his gall bladder in the morning. "Mr. Woodard, we'll be back in a few minutes." Dimino spoke to the Veteran.

"Sure, doc." The man, slated to have morning surgery, settled back for some serious television watching. The intern and I walked briskly to the nurse's station. Dimino went behind the counter. "What're you doing now?" I asked as the intern pulled open the chart of the patient we had just seen.

"I'm writing some orders on him." I hesitated for a minute or two while Paul wrote.

"You're writing orders before you fully examine the patient?"

"He's only a routine pre-op. Besides, if he needs anything else, I'll order it when I go back over him."

"Oh."

"If I wait till I finish, it may be twelve o'clock before any orders get written on him."

"Oh, that makes sense."

A few minutes more passed as Dimino finished writing the rest of the orders. "Now we got to go finish with Johnson."

A sudden realization changed my previous view of Mr. Johnson. If he was biting, fighting, and scratching when examined by the intern, he was likely to be considerably worse by the time I examined him. As we walked toward the old man's room, I tried ardently, and unsuccessfully, to think of a way for me not to do the admission.

We entered the room. Mr. Johnson was being cajoled by the sandy-haired nurse. I waited for him to strike as the intern and I approached.

"Mr. Johnson," the nurse said, "here are the doctors."

"Hello." Dimino shouted. "How are you feeling, Mr. Johnson?"

"Oh, just fine, doctor." He smiled pleasantly. I regarded him carefully.

"Mr. Johnson," Dimino continued to shout, "I'm going to examine you now."

"O.K., doctor." Dimino approached the old man, stethoscope in hand. Oh boy, here it goes. I braced myself for battle. There was none. The man who just half an hour before had been totally unmanageable was now fully cooperative. The power of Vitamin H, Haldol, was indelibly printed upon my mind.

Mr. Johnson was to teach me yet another lesson as my nose soon let me know. There was a distinct and unpleasant odor in the room which before had not been present. It was the smell of bloody stools, one of the hallmarks of bleeding from the intestine. Mr. Johnson, a ninety year-old former foot soldier who cursed like the proverbial sailor, had an unknown intestinal bleeding site. His hematocrit, a measure of the blood in his worn body, was twenty-eight, very low, and dropping. He was already getting blood and would need more.

The old man bore the intern's examination patiently, not complaining even as the rectal was being done. As Dimino completed his exam, he gave me leave to perform an abbreviated history and physical on the old man. As the intern's footsteps died in the hallway outside, I realized that I knew no short examination. Fortunately, Vitamin H, Haldol, continued working its tranquilizing and obscure magic.

CHAPTER 8

O God of surgery, cheater of Death, guide our steps so that we may deliver our charges safely from the Death-friend, Hemorrhage -
--Prayer of the priests of the God of the Knife

The priests of the God of the Knife did not want to operate. They wanted to avoid it at virtually any cost.

"It's Johnson ... "

"What's wrong. " I asked.

"He's bleeding again." Somewhere in Dimino's voice was reiterated the sentiment that no one wanted to operate on the 90 year old man.

"Where from?"

"I don't know. All I know is that his 'crit is dropping and he has black stools." Don't make us operate. You will *never make it off the table*. "Here . . . you type and cross him for some more blood. I'll put down the N. G. tube." Dimino passed me a tourniquet. He worked until evening when he signed out to Frank Payton, the intern who, with me, was on call. Throughout the night, Frank and I worked, transfusing blood, checking hemoglobins and hematocrits. I looked at the cooperative, yet, ornery old man who had survived a depression, a tour of active duty in France, dysentery, and seventeen VA - hospital admissions and whispered, please stop bleeding.

When the gray dawn entered through a part in the surgical green curtains, Mr. Johnson opened his eyes. We had reached a tenuous balance with the body of this gruff old man where the volume of blood we poured into him matched that which his body was pouring out.

"What's his "crit?" Joel appeared worn and mildly disheveled. I guessed the calls regarding Johnson's condition had been frequent throughout the night.

"Twenty-three. " I answered.

Joel appeared worried.

"We got to do something." Frank Payton who, along with me, had been on call and up most of the night spoke to the chief resident.

“I know." Joel answered.

“One more bleed like this and we can forget about it." Exasperation filled the intern's voice.

"I know.” Joel's face showed deep concern. "I don't want to operate on this guy. I'd better talk with the attending."

□ □ □ □

The vessels branching off the descending aorta were fresh in my mind after a brief review. I felt deep down dirty, grungy, after being up most of the night and having slept five minutes **too l**ong to catch the last remaining shower before rounds. Dimino, looking fresh and rested from a good night's sleep, pulled the front of the stretcher off the elevator. His black hair, parted in the center and cut to a length just above his ear, was neat and combed and his pants, usually wrinkled, were crisply pressed. Though I knew that as bad as were my nights on call, his were worse, though I knew that every human was entitled to one good night's sleep out of three, I knew also that I was tired and dirty and, yes, angry because I was those things and he was not. In the stagnated recording system of my mind a tape began to replay. An image of an old woman, hair whitened by the tread of years which had left her patient, loving, and only a little wrinkled, focused, faded, then focused again. "Doctor, how is he today?" she asked just as she had asked on many other occasions. I had come across her in the hall, feeding her husband patiently, a spoonful at a time, as if he were a new-born child unable to feed himself. "About the same, Mrs. Johnson. " I said, looking into eyes which oftentimes belonged to a gay young girl, but which would become clouded and tired when she began to ask me questions like these. I had realized that she was a better barometer of his well-being than any test, better than the combined clinical acumen of the entire team of physicians. She had - often known about changes in his condition hours before we were able to see it. As I was the only member of the team who spoke more than two sentences to her, questions like these were often her way of letting us know things had changed. I listened carefully to the spaces between sentences for any unsaid statements - There were none. She stepped toward me, out of earshot of her husband

The vessels branching off the descending aorta were fresh in my mind after a brief review. I felt deep down dirty, grungy, after being up most of the night and having slept five minutes **too l**ong to catch the last remaining shower before rounds. Dimino, looking fresh and rested from a good night's sleep, pulled the front of the stretcher off the elevator. His black hair, parted in the center and cut to a length just above his ear, was neat and combed and his pants, usually wrinkled, were crisply pressed. Though I knew that as bad as were my nights on call, his were worse, though I knew that every human was entitled to one good night's sleep out of three, I knew also that I was tired and dirty and, yes, angry because I was those things and he was not. In the stagnated recording system of my mind a tape began to replay. An image of an old woman, hair whitened by the tread of years which had left her patient, loving, and only a little wrinkled, focused, faded, then focused again. "Doctor, how is he today?" she asked just as she had asked on many other occasions. I had come across her in the hall, feeding her husband patiently, a spoonful at a time, as if he were a new-born child unable to feed himself. "About the same, Mrs. Johnson. " I said, looking into eyes which oftentimes belonged to a gay young girl, but which would become clouded and tired when she began to ask me questions like these. I had realized that she was a better barometer of his well-being than any test, better than the combined clinical acumen of the entire team of physicians. She had - often known about changes in his condition hours before we were able to see it. As I was the only member of the team who spoke more than two sentences to her, questions like these were often her way of letting us know things had changed. I listened carefully to the spaces between sentences for any unsaid statements - There were none. She stepped toward me, out of earshot of her husband.

“Do you think he's going to die?" She watched my face closely to see if it might betray a secret my lips would not.

“I don’t know.” I said as evenly as I could.

She scrutinized my features closely for a time. But it was true, I did not know. Her eyes welled as she moved toward a chair. I could see in her joints, knotted by arthritis, in her movements, aching and slow, that the years had left their mark. As she sat down, I offered her my handkerchief for I had nothing else to give.

"I'm sorry, doctor."

I fought the urge to tell her not to cry. "No, go ahead. There's nothing wrong with that." I said recalling the lesson I had learned in the office of a family physician, a priest of the Joined Hands.

She sobbed gently for a moment. "It's just that he's been sick for so long. I just don't know what to do." She stared into space for a time. "Every day I come, though it's hard. Thinking of her walking, I understood the difficulty of which she spoke. "It takes me two hours to get here and two hours to go home. I have to go home early or I won't be able to find a seat. I can't stand too long. I'm so worried that if he doesn't see me every day that he will just give up." Conviction, like a physical presence, hung heavily in the air. I felt angry at myself for being angry at Dimino. I felt angry at myself for succumbing to self-pity simply because I was tired and dirty, when some old lady hobbled on knees as old as dust just to give her husband lunch and the will to make it through one more day. The radiologist was talking. "One of you going to stay with him?" He looked at the intern.

"Yeah, he is." The intern looked at me. The radiologist looked at me, doubtfully.

I drew myself up proud and protective of my debilitated charge, this decrepit, weak, but still viable pile of humanity, with my full height, I looked the radiologist in the eye.

"Alright, then." He spoke to Dimino.

Grumfeld, the radiologist, was a stellar luminescence at an institution which boasted a host of academic stars. Each morning the priest with ever-tussled black hair and small, almost-beady eyes would call upon a priest-cadet, or resident-priest, or an intern to stand before a group of thirty priests-in-training. Depending upon the dictates of unmerciful caprice, the victim would be gently led down the paths of knowledge or driven by many pointed barbs into silent humiliation. The combination of Grumfel's unquestioned mastery of his field and his mercurial temperament caused the house staff to look forward to radiology rounds each morning with an odd mixture of joy and dread. *What was the priest's mood?* That was the question. I was certain that his fury would descend upon me at any moment for my gross impertinence. However, the priest who was neither young nor old, was in a strange mood. He went about the business of preparing the patient for the procedure silently. I decided to adopt an attitude of passive non-existence, a peculiar state often assumed by medical students, where one took on the posture of the nearest inanimate object and became as lifeless, quiet, and unobtrusive as that object. It was the last refuge, before flight, of those whose presence was required but not wanted. There was a great deal of moving the old man back and forth. Grumfeld left as the technicians continued with most of the preliminary work of setting the dials and positioning the patient.

□ □ □ □

"Everything ready?" Grumfeld re-entered the room.

"Yes." the technician answered. Grumfeld stood with his back toward me, facing the patient. "You ever see one of these before?" He half turned. It took a moment for me to realize that the priest was speaking to me. "No, I haven't."

"Are you planning to stay, or do you have to go to the floor?"

"No, I'm going to stay."

"Then you better put on an apron." I placed my arms through the holes in the plastic garment as I had seen the priest do. The weight of the over-sized kitchen apron surprised me as I lifted it onto my frame. Despite its weight, I had doubts about the protection it afforded. As the procedure got under way, however, I forgot these concerns.

"Where's the pedal," the priest called out.

"You got it right there by your right foot, Dr. Grumfeld."

"O.K., you want to turn that monitor a little more toward me." Grumfeld adjusted the overhead apparatus from which the x-ray beam emanated. "Everybody shielded?" He glanced around. He stepped on the pedal. All eyes went to the monitor where a series of undecipherable shadows appeared. The screen went blank before I saw a single recognizable structure. "we're too low." He moved the overhead apparatus up, toward the patient's head. The monitor lit up again. "Alright, we're in the right area now." The wire needs to come up some more. The resident in radiology who had been doing the procedure under Grumfeld's direction, pushed the catheter further into Mr. Johnson's groin. "Good. See the wire?" Grumfeld half-turned to me. I could see the vertebral column, the back bone. Anything else was a hopeless mass of undulating shadows. The priest read the uncertainty in my silence. "The wire's right there . . . Give me something to point with." Someone handed him a hemostat. "Right there." He pointed to a long shadow with a hook-like end which I realized was the image of the catheter in the Aorta, the body's main blood vessel. "Yes, I see it," I answered. The shadows began to take on forms with names that I knew. It was astounding. It was just like the anatomy which I had learned in the second year of medical school and which I had reviewed only moments before the procedure. The monitor went blank. "O.K., center it," Grumfeld called out. The overhead piece moved again. The catheter was in the aorta just below the diaphragm. A small patch of grayness indicated the opening to one of the major branches of the aorta, the coeliac artery which trifurcated into three major vessels.

"Easy, now." Grumfeld coaxed the resident. " . . . Easy. Not so fast." The catheter slipped past the opening to the coeliac. "Now, try again." Unsuccessfully, the resident tried several. More times. "Slowly, slowly . . . " The gray-black crook flitted past the opening again.

"I'm going to try, " Grumfeld said. The resident-priest stepped back. He handed the thin tube to Grumfeld, a tube which reached into the artery where my patient's life blood ebbed, drop by drop, as the grains of sand in an hour glass. The forces of the God of the Knife, locked in deadly combat with Hemorrhage, powerful servant of Death, were losing. Life in the old man was waning. Sensing victory for its master, Death, Sepsis could be heard approaching in the distance. John Johnson, perhaps aware of the closeness of his demise, perhaps too sick to care, remained silent. His usual complaints over every assault by the priests on his Body, his dry wit could not be heard. The frightened priest–cadet at the old man's side was being slowly inundated by a sea of hopelessness. It was, disquieting witnessing a battle which meant so much but which I could not actively join.

Say something, goddamit, you cantankerous old bastard, I thought.

"Shit." I did not know if he had heard my unspoken plea or if, in my agitation, I had shaken the table of which he lay, but my charge had spoken.

The opening of the coeliac continued to elude even the efforts of the attending-priest Grumfeld. "That's a tough one." No one answered. No one moved, Mr. Johnson complained of the hardness of the table.

"I know, Mr. Johnson - Try to be patient. It's important, " I patted the old man on the shoulder as I spoke.

He whispered an expletive not very softly. My attention returned to the monitor which blinked on . . . off . . . on, again and again. The room was becoming warm. Fatigue was etched across the faces of all in the room.

"Got it!"

"Alright." Bodies drew closer to the monitor. The coeliac and its three major divisions became visible. Grumfeld handed the catheter to the resident. The attending priest's eyes narrowed in concentration. I also studied the screen. Its familiar contours were lost to me once they entered the secondary branches - They were not laid out in textbook style as previously, but as one of the inconstant variations of real life. The foot pedal clicked at irregular intervals. Grumfeld spoke to the younger priest, prodding him to get a better view. The resident pushed, twisted, pulled the wire until the attending radiologist was satisfied. Both faces became again a mask of concentration.

"I think I see something there." Grumfeld spoke.

"Where?"

"Right there . . . coming off the left gastric. See if you can get some more dye down there." The resident obeyed.

"Let's test it. " The elder priest changed syringes once more. The gray column of contrast medium filled the hollow of the tube.

The catheter undulated with the old man's pulse. A gray column of grayness jumped forward into the blood stream. It did not move into the area where there had been bleeding previously. Instead, it moved from the order of the artery to the disorder of the capillary bed then, swiftly, back to the order of the vein.

"It seems to be holding."

*Yes."

"Let's try it again." All eyes turned to the monitor. The gray column returned to the former site of leakage and once more was repulsed by the thrombus.

"Alright, let's pull that catheter out of there." Each of the priests breathed a sigh of relief. "Sir," Grumfeld shouted, "you were really good during the procedure."

"Thank you." Mr. Johnson grunted

"Alright. Five minutes of direct pressure before he goes back." Grumfeld spoke to the resident. I stood near quietly as the resident priest pressed his thumb into the Old man's groin. Afterward, I pushed the stretcher slowly to the elevator and the fifth floor. Time, the true test of the success, showed that William Johnson's life-threatening bleeding had stopped. Soon his Bawdy language, dry wit, and cantankerous disposition returned, both to the amusement and consternation of the E Service.

CHAPTER 9

All priests are politicians. Some of us choose
to acknowledge this. Some of us do not.
--a priest of the God of Life

S**even: eight A.M**. I was breathless after a long rapid walk down the corridor.

"You're late!" Dr. Metcalf was angry. He was one of the attending-priests of the God of the Knife, a senior staff surgeon with features and mannerisms surprisingly boyish for his six decades. The students he dealt with daily he gave nick names like "sport", "slim". "Smiley" was the name he chose to call me in his more playful moods. As I smiled little, I do not know why he chose to call me that. "I had to wait for x-ray to open at seven. They wouldn't let me have the films overnight." I answered truthfully. "That doesn't cut any ice with me." His answer was curt.

Each priest of the cutting sect had his rules, often unfounded in science and illogical, but inviolate. The rules were perhaps a concession to a field of work controlled more by caprice than justice, a world where the best planned battle might be lost by casual and callous calamity. As each sect held sacred its God, each priest held sacred his rules. To violate the rule was to violate the priest. The resident-priests of the God of Surgery knew Metcalf's foremost rule well for several had lost an opportunity to practice the sacred cutting arts after arriving at the operating room late.

"You want to sit here by the blackboard?" Mark asked, as he made room for me to pass. I nearly tripped as I maneuvered to the far side of the cramped room. I spread the contents of the x-ray folder in front of me. Which one first? Yes, here it is. I shuffled the large pieces of plastic in the manila envelope as an over-sized deck of cards until I was satisfied with their order. The films were from one of my patients whose many clinical findings, including a heart on the wrong side of his body, had educated two generations of house officers. I cleared my throat. I glanced at my notes, a single sheet of notebook paper, on which I had written only the barest outline of my talk. My notes were only a reminder so that I would not omit any topic. I felt comfortable with my topic as I had studied well. I looked at my notes once more for confidence.

"The talk today is on pancreatitis." I was careful to look at each one of my classmates in turn as I spoke. I was determined that they were going to stay awake during my presentation. "What's the significance of pancreatitis? Under what circumstances might one see it?" I suppressed a grin as I recalled how many times I had been the audience of a similar gathering and had felt that these questions had been left unanswered even after two hours of lecture. Following up on the question, I described briefly how pancreatitis had to be considered in virtually every patient who presented with abdominal pain. Also, I told how pancreatitis could present as shock. I was surprised when I glanced at the clock and realized that I had been speaking continuously for twenty minutes. A head leaned slowly to the left, almost touching the one next to it. Pete Nathan's eyes were closed. He had been on call, up most of the night, sleeping less than two hours. Mark, who sat next to Pete, eyed the leaning head with annoyance as he pushed his elbow into Pete's side. Pete woke with a start. Mark, contented, returned his gaze to me. I felt sorry for Pete. We all knew, too well, what it felt like to be tired. Still speaking, I looked at Dr. Metcalf. He had missed the interaction between Mark and Pete.

A few minutes later the talk was concluded. Questions were asked, each of which I fielded easily and in depth. Metcalf asked a question which I answered at length.

"Alright, Smiley, that was a good talk." The attending-priest smiled. As the gathering broke up, a low growl escaped from my stomach. The freshly made coffee and donuts were more than welcome.

CHAPTER 10

In every religion there are those whose belief carry them into a world removed from this one, a world where the intensity of their devotion brings about a state of intense ecstasy, an uncontrolled trance state where the mind and body of the devotees become mere instruments of their God.

--Academy lectures

M**any times I had** witnessed the holy ire of the worshipers of the Knife which caused the priests' hands to shake. "Come on, Jim, let's go." The attending was becoming angry. The operation was taking much longer than it should have. There were no unexpected findings, no problems. The operator, James Trevor, a surgical resident one year beyond his internship, was slow. My stomach began to growl. I was grateful that through the three layers of clothing, the last aseptic, no one could hear. I was in a quiet, sedate mood, one which I had adopted many times since beginning the surgical rotation, one which I had often found myself in after pulling mindlessly at a retractor for the second hour running. At first, I would be bored, then angry, then I would lose tract of the surgery, drifting aimlessly over the canyons of my mind. Thoughts of many things past, recent and remote, would come to me. I would immerse myself in times and thoughts of silent, wistful brooding, but sometimes I would be carried away to happier times and a gentle smile would flicker behind my green surgical mask.

"Be careful with that." The attending priest indicated a piece of bowel which the resident was re-anastomosing. "No, not like that. Like this." Bond grabbed the needle holder from Trevor's hand. The attending priest placed several sutures. The young priest watched. Sadness and a new intensity covered his face.

"Here." Bond nearly threw the needle holder back at the resident. "Now, finish this."

There was virtually nothing to finish. The older priest had done almost the entire anastomosis. There was yet one more anastomosis to be done. The utter concentration, the devotion of the younger priest was undeniable. He's going to lose the case, I thought. Also, I knew that though I did exactly as instructed, fault would be found with me as well.

"Give me that." The older priest addressed me. He grabbed the retractor I was holding. I released the curved stainless steel blade. He re-positioned the instrument once, then, not satisfied, replaced it a second and a third time.

"Here." I took hold of the retractor. Its final position had not changed a single millimeter from the position it had held before Bond had wrested it from me. The young priest's hands, which before had exhibited a barely perceptible tremor, were noticeably shaking. Bond continued his harassment of the resident. I felt sympathy for Jim. He was an excellent teacher. Countless times he had taken a moment to explain an unclear point or to leave us, the student-priests, with a pearl. There were not many surgeons smarter than he and his patients found him warm and empathetic. But Jim was slow--an unforgivable flaw in a would-be surgeon. Each year thirty interns were accepted. Ten became residents. A year later only five continued and went on to finish the program.

Like so many surgical programs throughout the country, ours was pyramidal. Many were taken in, few finished. Jim was climbing the pyramid and losing. The holy ire overcame the resident-priest. His hands were markedly shaking as he moved within the full force of the holy trance state. Perhaps it was the hand of the God of the Knife which stayed Bond's anger. Perhaps it was the unabashed sincerity of the young devotee. I do not know. I know only that the young priest was allowed to finish the operation. At the close of the surgery, the holy ire which I had never understood, stood before me with unclouded clarity.

Its name was fear.

CHAPTER 11

The distinction between health and disease
is often one of patient perception.
--Academy lectures

It was as if my being resided in a gray metal sphere in which there was no light except a lone candle. Inside me was also devastatingly empty. I could call out to the walls which were not far distant. A single echo came as my only reply.

I was not at home within myself. I had hoped that others could fill the loneliness within me. I had hoped that others could give me the wholeness which I needed but which I was afraid to seek within myself. All another could do was to distract me, making me forget, for too short a time, the loneliness I carried within. Always when they were gone, and often, increasingly more often, while they yet remained, the loneliness haunted me as a relentless and unpitying ghost. I feared this void as I feared no human nor power on earth or beyond. It terrified me, causing my heart to race. It tortured me with an inhuman blend of psychic and physical pain. It took hold of me in the empty spaces between sentences. It occasioned strange looks as it seized me while I spoke and made me forget completely what I had been saying. Sometimes it seized me as I pedaled along the street or as I passed two lovers sharing an embrace. It often seized me during lectures or as I dreamed within a shallow sleep. I became afraid to dream. After a time, I was blessed with tiring, but dreamless sleep.

I was grateful for surgery. It allowed me to work long busy hours, as many as I wanted or needed. After a long day and evening, especially after being on call, I could throw myself onto the bed and fall headlong into the comforting arms of an undreaming sleep

CHAPTER 12

Tiredness and fear are the watch dogs of failure.

--bathroom graffiti, Academy of the Priests of God of Life

Surgery E. On call. Sunday. I made my way back down the long silent, linoleum-coated corridor to the pod which contained the sleeping quarters of the house officers. It was a slow day, filled with monotony and routine. I was a well-trained surgery medical student or "stud" as we were called. The work which was required of me, I knew. I did it quickly, quietly, efficiently. A dull slothfulness hung over me like sobriety to a man who wanted to get drunk but could manage neither inebriation nor forgetfulness. My mood allowed no effective reading. My footsteps sounded empty echoes as I turned the last corner. The sound of television greeted me. A football game was on. I followed the sound to the largest of the on-call rooms which contained five beds. Dausman looked up at my coming. Across his face was a large boyish grin which belied the appearance of age conferred on him by the bald spot he tried half-heartedly to hide. I felt comfortable around Dausman. I seldom felt this in the presence of my fellow medical students. Also, I liked his sense of humor. I turned my attention to the television program.

"What've you been doing all day?" he asked.

"A whole lot of nothing. Nothing exciting. What about you?"

Ernie turned toward me. "We had a couple of admissions earlier. I was hanging out in the E.R. for a while. A few interesting cases came. Some guy came in with nasal bleeding. I got to pack his nose."

"That's pretty good."

"You want to watch something else? I'm not watching this. "

"No, that's O.K."

"There's nothing else better on. How're things going? You really look tired."

"No. Just bored. You know I really hate being on call on Sunday."

"Yeah, I know. It really sucks. Sure you don't want to watch something else?"

"No, I'm O.K."

"How do you like working with Gail Reed?" He leaned toward me. I said nothing while trying to suppress a smile. "I can't stand that disgusting little winch."

We both laughed. I was only able to tolerate her by ignoring her existence. Though we had never spoke of Gail, Dausman had obviously known.

"Come on, tell the truth. You can't stand her either."

"We-ell . . ." We both laughed heartily again.

"I can't stand the way she's always kissing up to the attendings. And she's so frigging ugly." Dausman had me laughing despite myself.

"Guess who she's going out with?"

It was difficult to think of anyone being attracted to Gail. "Who?"

"Mark Polsky."

"Oh, come on."

" I swear. You think I'm lying."

"Oh, come on, Ernie."

"No, it's the truth. Pete Nathan saw them together."

I shook my head in disbelief. I spoke aloud. "I wonder what they do together."

"Probably discuss surgery. What else could you do with an ugly broad like that."

We laughed again. "You know, Mark is such a god damn nice guy, but he's so square."

"Really?"

"Yeah, and he's so smart he makes me look like a schmuck."

"Oh, yeah?"

"You know, he goes home every night and stays up to midnight reading. He really loves this stuff. He wants to go into surgery, probably ENT."

"I didn't know that."

"You don't have anything to worry about. You seem to know this stuff pretty well."

"I don't know about that."

"You're going into surgery too, aren't you?" A piercing high-pitched noise broke the air. I followed Ernie's hand to the box at his side. A static-ridden voice told Ernie what number to call.

"You got a beeper?" I asked incredulously.

"Yeah, they give us one on D service." He tried to answer nonchalantly, but was as successful as I was at disguising my obvious envy. I watched as he dialed the number. He chatted amicably for half a minute then hung up the phone.

"You got to draw blood or something?"

"No, he just wanted to know where I was."

"Oh."

Dausman sighed. "It's so dull around here. I should be reading, but I can't read anymore. You get any reading done?"

"No, not much." Mild, very mild, feelings of guilt jogged across my consciousness.

"Where's your team? I haven't seen them much today."

"I don't know. I think Arnie's sleeping. I don't know where Joel is." I looked at the television screen, only vaguely aware of what was going on. It was a comedy which Dausman enjoyed very much. My thoughts drifted first to the topic of a breakfast conference in two days. The topic was one I knew little about and would require my seeking information from several sources. My mind began to wander further, as it often did in idle moments to Grace. This was the major reason that I tried to keep my unoccupied time to a minimum. Where was she? There was a dry hardness in my throat as I thought with whom she might be. Perhaps Lance, that shadowy figure whose path by some odd dictate of chance never crossed mine. What might they be doing? I followed their images in my mind until they were naked together in a

lover's embrace. The sound of ecstasy saturated my pores and came to rest in the emptiness of my intestines. A voice, my own, bade me stop.

"Where are you going?"

I called back over my shoulder to Dausman. "I have to check on a few things. See you."

"See you."

My footsteps resounding in the hall carried the air of hurried importance. I slowed down. What did I have to do? Where was my team? I had not seen them for a while.

"There you are." Joel's voice surprised me. I had not seen him until he spoke.

"Hi"

"Bond's coming in. We're going to do a portal-caval shunt." The words denoted several hours of intense surgery. The operation, for which the chairman of the Department of Surgery was well-known, was an all out effort to save the life of a person whose liver was little more than a fibrous band. Usually the person had a history of bleeding from the upper intestine.

"A G.I. Bleeder?" I asked the chief resident.

"Yes."

"Esophageal varices?"

"Yep."

I began to try and guess my position during the procedure. Kelly, the chairman, as well as our own attending, Bond, would be there. With Joel and the intern also scrubbed that left me either nothing or the dreaded "brown mole" position. (This position derived its name from the brown mole on the back of the chairman's neck which was all of the operation the occupant was allowed to see while pulling steadfastly on a retractor.

The chief resident turned to leave then stopped.

"What're you doing now?"

"I was going to check on some labs."

"Do what you can, then let Schom finish the rest. I want you scrubbed on this case."

"Sure." I beamed. At least there was a chance that I would see some of the operation.

"You'll be second assistant."

"Second assistant?!"

"Yeah. Bond, me and you will be scrubbed."

"What about Arnold?"

"He'll be on the floor taking care of patients." This was more than I had even dreamed. Me, a third year medical student, barely on the wards a month, second assisting on an operation that few besides the priests of the Knife would ever see. It was too much. The hours of boredom were an evanescent memory. I turned to go, then stopped short.

"How long before he goes to surgery?"

"An hour."

"Alright, see you then."

"O.K." he called over his shoulder.

Now to find Dausman. I wanted him to see the shunt and share my good fortune.

□ □ □ □ □

The sound of the water running furiously, futilely, into the stainless-steel sink reminded me of the sound one heard inside a car that was being pulled through a car wash. The running water was an unnecessary waste, I felt. When scrubbing alone and not in the presence of the priests, I turned the water off while I lathered my arms and hands. As Joel was present, my water ran without pause. Joel was in a good mood. More than this, he was in a teaching mood. He reviewed the procedure at length which I was about to see. More and more as time passed, he took me aside, instructing me in the rites of the priesthood. This he did with me much more than any of the other students of my class.

Dausman approached as I stood at the sink with the chief resident.

"Hi, Ernie."

"Hi." Dausman pulled down a betadine saturated sponge and turned on a tap. I knew Joel would not object to Ernie watching. I did not know how he would feel about Ernie scrubbing.

"You're scrubbing on this operation?" Joel asked the question evenly.

"Yeah." Dausman answered.

"Good." The chief resident continued his discussion. The patient, whom I saw for the first time as I entered the operating room, was sinking into the last stages of the death-like artificial sleep of anesthesia. The orange color of his skin was apparent even in the unnatural light of the operating room. Norm took his position at the patient's side. Dausman and I moved to the opposite side of the patient.

"May we begin?" Joel looked at the anesthesiologist.

"Yes, he's ready."

"Knife." A stainless-steel scalpel was placed in the chief resident's hand. A band of yellow-white fat appeared as the blade glided over the man's skin. "Beginning my incision." The circulating nurse glanced at the clock. It was midnight.

"I'm going to hang some more blood." The anesthesiologist spoke to Joel.

"Yeah, go ahead. Which unit is that for him?"

"The fourth."

"How many more does he have?"

"He's crossed for six more."

The door opened and swung closed. Bond's nasal tone asked "Where are you?"

"I'm opening peritoneum."

The surgeon's hands were covered with brown foam. "What's his last 'crit?"

"Twenty-eight." The room was almost silent.

"It's probably really more like twenty."

"Yeah."

The attending-priest went back outside. He finished his scrub quickly. As he returned to the operating table, the two student-priests were shuffled to different positions leaving Ernie in the dreaded right upper quadrant position. This was like the brown mole position except that its occupant was able to see the beginning of the surgery. With the arrival of the second surgeon, the operation began in earnest.

Soft pink intestine was packed out of the way with half a dozen lap pads. Each pad had a large metal ring attached to it which remained outside the patient. The operation proceeded. It became clear why the position held by Dausman was so disliked. Virtually none of the surgery was visible to Ernie. As it neared three o'clock, his eyes were bathed in the dull focuslessness of the peri-somnolent. I cleared my throat to wake Ernie. He remained in the semi-sleep state. I cleared my throat again, hoping he would hear me. I could think of nothing to say which would not give him away. I cleared my throat a third time.

"What's the matter, you got a cold or something?" the attending-priest asked.

I could not remember if one could scrub with a cold. I had to answer. "No, just clearing my throat."

Both priests continued to look into the abdomen. Ernie looked at me, not comprehending what was taking place, but at least awake. Intermittently, I looked up at Ernie. Half the time he was sound asleep. I cleared my throat a lot.

"Don't toe in that blade!" Joel spoke to Ernie. I looked at Ernie. He was teetering like a felled oak. He edged forward at an increasingly faster rate. Oh, no, he's going to fall right into the operating field. There was no time to call out.

Wham! Dausman's descent into the patient's intestines was stopped abruptly by a gut-wrenching elbow into his mid-section. Ernie startled awake. I looked at Joel who had un-gently awakened the student-priest. His eyes had not left the field. I looked at Bond. He seemed not to have noticed the incident. Once again before the procedure was finished the student-priest headed downward into the operating field and was checked by the chief resident's elbow. I fully expected to see a second set of intestines spewed across the room. My colleague stood upright, annoyed, but intact.

□ □ □ □

A few days later.

"Ernie, I'm really sorry about that operation."

"What operation?"

"The portal-caval shunt."

"Oh, that."

"Yeah, I thought you were going to watch. I didn't intend for you to get stuck holding back the liver."

"Don't worry about it?"

"Hey, but I really feel bad."

"Hey, it's O.K." Though Dausman did not blame me, I felt bad

nonetheless. I did not ask Ernie to see an "interesting case" again.

CHAPTER 13

All Gods in the House of Life serve the God of Life.

--Credo of the Priests of the God of Life.

Bond sat back calmly; the two tails of his long white coat drawn over his long thin legs. The blue empty space of his eyes regarded us with contained anticipation. I watched my classmates. Mark Polsky, smooth walnut hair and pleasant angular features which made him look as if he were smiling even during the rare times he was not. I liked Mark. Gail Reed's nose turned upward at the end, giving her otherwise unremarkable face an appearance which alternated between that of an agreeable elf and a sandy-haired sorceress. She watched the attending priest from a minute, self-contained corner. Dausman chewed his nails as perspiration made his bald spot shine. Bond tossed questions at us through the steel-rimmed frames of his glasses in a voice perennially nasal. A low pitched, dissatisfied growling escaped from my belly managing, through three layers of clothing, to dispel the quiet. I drew my arms closer around my abdomen and swallowed all too audibly.

Even the never-ending drone of hospital activity paused noticeably as the priest reflected. The blueness of his eyes narrowed just the minutest bit as he threw a question gently, surprisingly gently, toward us. We student-priests were wary. The God of the Knife was not a generous God. Any gift so easily received was suspect. Each of us expected a trap. Each of us examined the question for an unbelievable long silent space of time.

I looked at our examiner. His expression said that he was neither lying nor trying to trick us. I did not trust him. My classmates felt likewise. After the grueling weeks we had spent under the tutelage of the priests of the Sanguine God, we suspected that the question was a trick, one which would turn treacherously on any fool enough to touch it. The expressions of my fellow students were those of plastic mannequins steeled for the verbal flogging that would come if no one answered the question. They obviously preferred the berating for saying nothing to that for a wrong answer. I tossed the question in my mind yet another time, searching for hidden meanings, unnoticed nuances. There were none. I was determined to do well on surgery, no matter what. I answered the question. At first my voice was faltering and unclear. Soon it rose in both clarity and conviction. If I was to make an ass of myself it would not be because I stuttered. Bond's voice betrayed only the barest hint of surprise as he regarded me. I smiled as he acknowledged to the amazement of all four student priests, that I was right. The priest was taken aback further when I answered the next several questions as well. Though he was the surgery E attending I had never said much on our routine rounds with him. Often, he held rounds with only the chief resident. When the entire team was present it was clear that the medical students were expected to remain silent.

The questions grew more difficult. Ernie and Gail appeared relieved when I answered a question. Mark seemed reluctant to venture an answer about which he was not absolutely sure. Questions continued with increasing speed.

Some I did not know. Most of the time neither did my classmates. When preceptor rounds were over, I had answered almost three quarters of the questions.

Doubt lingered with me. Had the questions all been tricks and I not wise enough to hear the ringing laughter of the priest? It was not until the following week, when the attending priest actually spoke to me and smiled that I realized that I had passed yet another secret test of the God of the Knife.

CHAPTER 14

"There's more bootie on the ward than you can shake a stick at."
--an unnamed student-priest

When I started on the wards, I went through a blanking period. I could not remember a patient's name. I could not remember the name of a single house officer. Indeed, if my own name had not been affixed to my name tag, I would have forgotten it as well. I did not recognize faces during this time. So many ghosts drifting so swiftly before me scared me.

She was not a ghost. I had no trouble remembering her face. Caramel brown, attractive, with the smiling cheeks I always loved on any woman. She was tall, large-boned with only slightly nicely thick hips and two large dots for breasts. Her name I did not know for weeks. When finally, I heard it, it was quickly forgotten.

Near the end of my first rotation at the V.A., I began to feel more comfortable in my new surroundings. I realized that my legs would not fall off from standing, that every person passing in the hall was not jotting down notes for my evaluation, that I would not fold under what I considered an enormous workload, that I would make no mistake that would kill anyone. In short, I learned my place among the scheme of things on the wards. I raised my head above the over-magnified, muddled pond of hospital life. I realized that there was a world outside the concrete castle which trained white coated warriors. I realized that that world went on quite well without me whether or not I read a newspaper once a week to acknowledge its existence. I realized that despite my attempts at putting the shambles of a broken marriage out of my head I needed female companionship. More than this, and perhaps more urgently, I knew that though my tired body craved sleep, the stirring in my pants at odd hours of the day and night told me that I needed a woman's body more.

"There's more stuff on the wards than you can handle," a senior medical student had told me in my freshman year. His activities at a week-long conference during which we shared a room, made me believe that he spoke from experience. I had been then living with my wife and was interested in no other woman. Yet the comment had stayed in my mind. I'll be hot stuff when I get to the wards, I had thought. Even as my colleague spoke these words, a question gnawed at the edges of my consciousness. Why weren't the women falling over me already? I had placated myself by saying that it was because I was married.

I began spending more time on 5-East where the tall, brown-skinned ward clerk worked. I suggested that we have lunch together. She agreed, a smile blossoming upon her lips. As she returned to her desk with what I imagined was an extra little twist in her hips for me, I realized that I did not know her name. I was still in my forgetful stage.

□ □ □ □

She arrived with a girlfriend for lunch. Her friend's presence relieved me of the obligation to make the subtle and not so subtle come-ons, the suave remarks which I would have felt compelled to at least attempt. Though I was grateful that her friend called her name, conversation seemed to flow more easily when Karen and I were alone. We spoke briefly about several things, including discos. Dancing sounded like fun. I asked Karen out Friday.

THE THIRD YEAR

CHAPTER 15

Remember always that the power of priests
is the power of consent.
--Academy lectures

Thursday night I was on call. At six-thirty P.M. on Friday, after working all but four of the previous thirty-five hours, I hung up my coat and headed for the elevator. As always when I left before midnight, I felt an inexplicable twinge of guilt. I searched the worn cogs of my memory. Was there something I had forgotten? The answer was no. Still I looked around me furtively as I made my way toward the elevator. I pressed the button. Footsteps approached. The doors opened. I stepped quickly inside. The footsteps passed without revealing my presence. Once home, I was barely able to take off my clothes before falling headlong into a deep sleep.

□ □ □ □

I awoke, pouncing upon the alarm clock. I swore. The dial confirmed that it was time to get up. Sleep, a persistent lover, demanded at least another half-hour from my body. Forty-five minutes later I got up. Hurriedly, I began gathering my clothes. Casual was the mood. As I came out of the shower, I noticed that there were only twenty minutes left before I was to pick up Karen. There was no way I could make it.

I picked up the phone.

"Hello."

"Hello, Karen?"

"Un-huh." She sounded as if she were stretching.

"I'm going to be a few minutes late. About fifteen minutes or so."

"O-ka-a-ay." She was still stretching.

□ □ □ □ □

Her apartment was surprisingly sparsely furnished. Besides an impressive stereo, only a few lonely pieces of furniture distilled the room's emptiness. The acrid smell of marijuana was carried through the still air. Karen sucked on a small flattened brown cigarette.

"Want some?" She extended the glowing ember to me. I said nothing for the space of half a second.

"Do you smoke?" She asked.

"No, I don't." I tried to sound as hep as I felt square at that moment.

"I just do it once in a while," she intimated. "I'll be with you in a minute." She walked into the kitchen exuding a subtle sensual rhythm which neither promised nor denied, which was a statement of her own comfort with her body. The perceiver was left to make whatever message he could out of her motion. As I half lay, half sat before the speaker, the record player drove out a tune which I had never before heard. Before the night was over, the melody would accompany me to sleep.

Karen's daughter was at the home of her co-worker. She wanted to stop there briefly before going to the club. As we made our way to the house, she attempted to dictate every detail of my driving. Trying hard to keep this minor annoyance minor, I wondered would my hopes for a sterling night be realized.

□ □ □ □ □

The Backway was jumping. We headed for the bar. Most of the people were doing a step with which I was unfamiliar. After half a margarita, I did not care. I pulled my date on to the floor. Karen had told me that the name of this place had been Dance Your Rump Off. That's exactly what I did.

CHAPTER 16

It is important for priests-in-training to have the experience of being on call. It is equally important that they be off call. The optimal management of work, family, and leisure time and the maintenance of adequate quantities of each is a perennial dilemma which faces practicing priests throughout their careers.

--a priest of the God of the Joined Hands

T**hough the heat** was oppressive, I did not sweat. Karen's forehead and cheeks were beaded with perspiration. As we danced, she looked as a flower about to welter. A television camera swept by us. A whirling jumble of indistinguishable figures passed across the screen. The record ended. Karen pushed toward the bar where her purse and our drinks lay.

Water flowed in small quick streams down her face. I did not try to keep her on the floor as I had for the previous three records.

"Are y'all ready to pa-a--ar-tay?" The disc jockey screamed over the loud speaker.

"Yeah!" a solid chorus answered.

"I can't hear you. Are y'all ready to PAR-TAY?!"

"YEAH!"

"Alright then. Let's party." A guitar slid into some heavy funk.

"Are you all right?" I asked Karen. She looked faint.

"Huh?"

The music was loud. I leaned closer to her. "Are you all right?"

"I'm O.K."

I looked at her doubtfully. "Why don't we go get some air?"

"I'm O.K." She clutched her purse. She looked over the dance floor with an air of forced casualness. I felt that she was trying to convince me that she was all right. I did not press her.

As we stood at the bar a young man came up to Karen and began a conversation. It seemed as if Karen knew him. Two other guys had done this previously.

"You come here often?" I asked when the man had left.

"Sometimes." she answered coyly. "When I first moved to Canon, I used to come here a lot."

"Yeah. I noticed you seem to know quite a few folks here."

"Yeah." She was wearing that coy smile again. I wanted to get back on the dance floor. I decided to wait another record to allow my date to recover fully.

The hands of the clock in the corner were approaching twelve-midnight. A brief outline of the coming day was sketched in my mind. Get up at five for rounds at six-thirty. I was already dragging from staying up till two-thirty Thursday night when I had been on call. After work rounds in the morning at the V.A. was Grand Rounds at the U. from eight to twelve. Then try to get exercise, shopping, and rest before reporting for call at seven on Sunday morning. It was an impossible task, I knew. No matter what I did, I would be dragging in the morning on rounds and I would still be dragging Sunday when I reported for work.

What else was new? The disco took a sudden turn toward infectious funk. I wanted to move.

"Can I have this dance?" A man's hand was extended before me. My heretofore wilted date placed her hand in his and moved smilingly to the dance floor. I was crushed. She had discussed this with me beforehand. "You don't mind if I dance with someone else, do you?" she had asked.

"No," I had tried to answer matter-of-factually. "I'm sure you'll do the same," she had said graciously. Still, as she was led away, I was left with the feeling that I had lost something.

I leaned against the bar attempting to look a practiced suave. At times I would catch sight of my date. She seemed to be watching me often as well. As the record ended, she took two steps and then was pulled back on the floor.

She eyed me discretely as she moved in time to the music. I wandered from the bar to an area where several women watched the floor. Most sat in groups without men. I looked over them carefully, my eyes finally coming to rest on a woman sitting with two girlfriends whose smooth dark skin spoke of a regal richness.

She had as attractive face and wore a white cotton top which accentuated her more than ample breasts. Faded blue jeans hugged her thin waist and generous hips. I saw, or imagined I saw, an "I'm available" look as she saw me. The record was changing. I moved toward her. From nowhere, a hand reached out, pulling her on the floor. Foiled again.

I pulled a tall slender woman onto the floor. As we danced, Roberta and I exchanged names, nothing else. I saw the beautiful girl with deep brown eyes and pretty, dark skin several times. However, after Roberta and I ended our dance I saw her no more. She had vanished.

I returned to the bar and waited several records for my date. I caught up with her four records and twenty minutes later. Slave was on the turntable with "Slide", the deliciously wicked tune that had been on Karen's stereo.

Another and another record followed. We still danced. Higher and faster I danced. All the dancers were exhausted. The D.J. read the crowd well. He laid down a sensuous, soft, eminently slow danceable tract. I held Karen for yet another dance. Holding her, moving slowly across the floor, feelings were aroused which I tried to suppress. I was attracted to Karen. My feelings for her were those of a man for a woman.

I looked into her expressionless face which neither invited nor rejected. I decided to enjoy the movement of the record, the dim lights, and the closeness if only for one record. As the record ended, we walked slowly off the floor.

CHAPTER 17

"I'm a doctor."
"So?"
"I'm a doctor."
"So what?"

--recurring nightmare of a student priest

The hour of two A.M. and closing time drew near. The night had been a very pleasant diversion. I was again waiting for my date to return. Record followed record. As I stood at the edge of the dance floor, a tall, heavily-built, but not fat, woman asked me to dance. Several records began and ended as we moved to unrelenting sound. The woman became drunk with the driving rhythm, the screaming D.J., and the wall-to-wall body contact. During a particularly frenzied piece she threw her arms around my neck. I continued dancing though feeling considerably ill at ease.

"After this, one more record . . . Only one more record after this." The D.J. shouted to the crowd. "You Brothers better start getting some phone numbers if you don't want to spend the night alone." We laughed. I thanked my partner for the dance. I owed my date the last dance.

I waited patiently where Karen had left her purse. The last record began its introduction. Connie danced nearby with a man in a navy-blue leisure suit. As she moved toward the bar, he caught her hand and they began again. I felt slighted.

Quickly, I looked around for a partner, but saw only men who, like me, wanted someone with whom to dance. As I looked from the side lines, I felt desperate, frightened, sad, and lonely.

The music ended. People, mostly young men alone or in small groups, poured into the street. Karen was stopped several times on her way out by friends, all of whom were male. The weariness of the previous night on call began to wear on me. My mind began to wander back to my morning duties. After polite introduction, I waited impatiently while Connie spoke with her friends.

"There's another party at Crosstown." she told me as we walked toward the car.

"Oh, really?" I was doing a poor job of covering a yawn.

"Yeah, it's supposed to be really good."

I said nothing. After seeing the disinterested look on my face, she added testily. "You're not too tired, are you?"

"We-ell," I said trying to suppress a rising anger, "I have early rounds in the morning. I think I had better get at least a couple hours of rest."

"O.K., let's go." She made no attempt to hide her chagrin.

We traveled the three to four miles to her house in ten minutes. I pulled into an empty space in front of her building. I felt like a little conversation and perhaps a good night kiss. I had cooled down and felt that she had as well.

I cut the engine off. The white head beams went dark.

"Well, it was an interesting night." I said in my best mellow suave voice, as I leaned familiarly toward her.

"Yeah, I hope you had fun." she said as she opened the door. I nearly fell into her empty seat. Quickly, I opened my door. "I'll see you to your door."

She was already several yards away. "No, that's O.K. Good night." she called without looking back.

"Good night."

She was already out of sight. The door slammed. The cloak-like quiet of west Isle Street seemed alive with the buzzing electricity of the Backway. The searing beats ran through my body with an unquenchable excitement. Even the fingers of ever-faithful sleep, could not still the rhythms which lulled me to my rest. Awaking at the usual time, I swore less than the usual number of curses, and took less than the usual time to stumble into the bathroom. In the shower I scrubbed viciously to remove the telltale marks left on a man who had come home without even a good night kiss.

A grim face stared back at me from the mirror. Suddenly, I began laughing heartily. I was still alone and still had the aching in my loins, but I had come away with something that I had not had for even longer than it had been since I had had a woman--a good time. My heart felt strangely less burdened as I traveled to work with the red-gold sun gilding the road before me.

CHAPTER 18

We fight for the soul of a priesthood founded by the knowledge our ancestors and whose skills are honed on the suffering of their descendants.

--A priest of the Semi-Secret Society of Priests of the God of Life

The student grape vine was filled with stories of Ed Rind, the chief resident of Urology. None of the accounts were good.

I was eating lunch at the U. across from me sat two of my classmates, Rich Picard and Patrick Stein.

"What are you doing next?" I asked Pat. He looked up from a tuna salad sandwich.

"General Surgery at the V.A." A garbled southern accent was discernible between chews. "What about you?"

I took a bite of my only moderately dry hamburger garnished with ketchup and warm grease. "Urology," I answered. Both Pat and Rich erupted in laughter. Pat almost choked.

"You're taking Urology?" Pat recovered quickly. I eyed the two curiously over the edge of my quickly disappearing hamburger. Dry and plain or not, I was hungry.

"Yeah," I answered as I took another bite.

"Rich is taking it now."

"Oh man, you're in trouble." Rich leaned over the table.

"Yeah?"

"I'll never be so glad to leave a place in my life."

"Rich had a fight with the chief resident."

"A real physical fight." Rich added.

"So, I heard." Dausman had told me this earlier, but I had discounted the tale as being gross exasperation. Listening to Rich himself, I still found it hard to believe that Rich, whose face was that of a choir boy, had gotten into a fight with anyone. I had always been struck with what had seemed the gentleness of his character. The aggressiveness which was almost universal among my classmate and which seemed to be a prerequisite for entrance into medical school was nowhere evinced in him. What on earth could cause Rich to fight anyone? My hamburger finished, I listened attentively.

I was sitting I the radiology conference room. Ed comes in with the rest of the guys and says “That’s my chair.” There are about ten chairs around. All of them the same. “That’s my chair. I always sit there”

Then he starts pushing me out of the chair like I'm a bag of grocery or something."

"You're kidding!"

"No, I'm not. So, we're there pushing each other back and forth. I thought we were going to start punching each other until the others broke it up and he got another chair."

"Jesus Christ!"

"The whole thing was so incredibly stupid."

"Can you believe that?" Stein had finished the tuna salad sandwich.

"I got to really do well the next six weeks at the V.A. They're going to give me a lousy evaluation, I know."

I agreed.

CHAPTER 19

Success and perseverance are born of the same womb.

--Precepts of the Semi-Secret Society

Burns was the topic of the weekly surgical conference which had taken me away from the University Hospital. Burns were dull when compared to the most interesting consult the urologists had had in months. I returned to 3-East as work rounds were beginning.

Fred Noonan, the junior urology resident, quizzed Ed Rind. "How come you didn't incise the one across the top?" Fred and Ed had seen the consult.

"What did you find when you examined this guy?" Matt, the fellow on urology, had not seen the patient. Though Matt outranked Ed, he involved himself little in the day to day running of the service. He left this to Ed.

Ed's eyes widened. "There were these rings just sitting there, sticking out of this guy's penis."

"Rings?" Matt asked. "What kind of rings?"

"You know, those rings that you put through notebook paper?"

Matt looked puzzled.

"You know," Ed explained, "the ones that open up in the center and you stick 'em in the holes for the three-ring kind of notebook paper." Ed used his best Brooklyn-ese.

"Oh, yeah."

"Well those things were sticking in this mass of infected tissue."

"Did he put them all the way through or what?" Matt wanted all the details. I nudged closer as we walked down the hallway.

"No, he just put them in a half inch or so. Looks like he kind of just burrowed into the flesh." At this point Ed made a twisting motion with his fingers like turning a key in a lock, but more forceful. It made me only slightly nauseous.

"What did it look like?"

"There were these necrotic draining sinuses."

"There was all kind of necrotic debris and pus." Fred interjected.

"Yeah, it had the foulest odor and was the nastiest thing you ever saw. You can't believe the stuff that came out of there."

"So, what did you do?"

"I cleaned it up with some betadine and then I took a kelly and pulled them out."

"Did you use local?" Matt wanted to know if Ed had numbed the area first.

"No, why?"

"Didn't it hurt him?"

"No, more than it did when he put 'em in." There was a perverse, but undeniable, logic to this statement. I watched as Ed's hands followed a familiar pattern from pocket to pocket until he found a cigarette.

"How come you didn't incise the one on top." Fred's question would not be denied.

Ed lit a cigarette. He turned to look at the junior resident while he sucked on the glowing white stick. He began in a tone which was both condescending and sarcastic.

"What are you going to accomplish by that?"

"Help drainage."

"The damn thing had two well-formed sinus tracts already from the goddamn rings. It didn't need any more drainage sites." He sucked on the cigarette again.

"What did you do with him after that?" Matt asked the chief resident.

"Put him on antibiotics and gave him an appointment for clinic in a couple of days."

"The psych people see him?"

"Yeah, they're the ones who called the consult to us."

"They going to keep him?"

"Yeah, I guess so."

"He peeing O.K.?

"Yeah, yeah."

"Hmp." Matt looked bewildered. "Why'd he do it?" His mid-western accent rang clearly.

"Wanted to get rid of it." We stood before the door which led to the stairwell.

"Why'd he want to do that?" Matt asked.

"'Cause he couldn't get any."

"'Cause he couldn't get laid?" Matt shook his head.

"Jesus Christ!" Fred's voice came from behind. "Didn't he ever hear that guys with rings in their peckers don't score?"

We all roared. Our laughter could be heard over the flights of stairs as the door closed behind us.

CHAPTER 20

You can tell urologists by their yellow shoes.
--a saying of the priests of
the House of Life

I **had elected to** spend the morning helping the intern, Munger, with ward chores, "skut", as it was called in the jargon of house staff. All the other urologists were in the operating room. The cases were those in which I would have been relegated to a second-tier post from which I would have seen only the backs of the priests of the yellow shoes. Much of the surgery of urology fell into this category. Chuck was glad for the extra hand. I was glad to be doing something productive.

There was an increase in the usual activity inside the conference room. The room also served as a nurse's lounge and reading room. The morning wore on uneventfully. The door to the conference room opened frequently, but always closed before revealing the secrets within. The nurses and aids chatted happily as they passed within and without the room. Between the passings which were always carried out with amicable stealth, I was able to glean the gradual assembly of a feast far beyond any I had ever seen at the University

Hospital. My mouth watered. I thought of the dried hamburger which I usually had for lunch. I sighed, then returned to the work I had to do. No need day dreaming.

Cheryl's hand, protruding from a puffy yellow satin sleeve, glided almost effortlessly as she wrote. I do not believe that I ever saw Cheryl sit still for more than the space of a few seconds except on the rare occasions when she actually took her break. Even as she spoke of nothing in particular, she worked. I stood at Cheryl's desk, making small talk as Munger approached. As the intern drew near, she stiffened withdrawing completely into her work.

"Any problems?" he asked me.

"No, no problems."

He seemed relieved. I often was silently amused by his concern regarding the few uncomplicated tasks he gave me. He did not know that I had worked at a much higher level of function on Surgery E. Mainly, I wrote orders for various lab tests which he co-signed. I also wondered what kind of students had passed through urology before me.

The intern looked at his watch, then shook his head. He started off.

"What's the matter?" I asked.

He turned. "I wanted to see that nephrectomy." He seemed sad. "By the time I get down there, the case will be just about over."

"What do you have to do?"

"Draw bloods on three patients and change a foley."

"That's all."

"Yeah."

"Leave them for me, Chuck."

"I don't want to dump all the work on you. Besides, you already have work to do."

"I'm just about finished the stuff you gave me. All I have to do now is finish writing out this consult."

He looked at me doubtfully. "I don't know. The blood drawers weren't able to draw Metcalfe."

There was one thing I knew I could do--draw blood.

"Chuck, I'll get the blood."

"You sure?"

"I'm sure."

"Well, O.K. Thanks a lot." He flashed a grateful smile, then hurried toward the elevator.

Cheryl spoke to me. She had neither raised her head from her charts nor acknowledged the intern's presence in any way. "You know, I can't stand him."

I chuckled. Chuck had espoused a similar sentiment toward Cheryl.

"You're coming to our party, aren't you?" She looked into my face.

As I answered, I tried hard to keep the outpouring of saliva from the corners of my mouth from betraying my anticipation. "0-oh. That's what's going on in the conference room. Well, if you're inviting me . . . "

"Of course, you're invited," she insisted. "And don't tell me you're going to eat any of that cafeteria food either."

She paused long enough for me to accept the invitation.

"I'll be glad to come. Thank you."

"Alright, then. Whenever you get some time you just go on in there and help yourself."

"O.K., I have a few things I have to do first."

"O.K., then." She returned to her work as I went to the clean utility room.

The work Munger had given me took me forty minutes. The time passed quickly as I darted from one room to the next. I approached the nurse's station. I reached over Cheryl for lab slips as she worked at her desk. She took the lab slips from me before I could stamp them.

"No, let me do that." She placed the multi-colored pieces of paper beneath the addressograph. "What do you want on these?"

"A CBC, 'lytes, BUN, and creatinine."

"O.K." she answered as she checked off the boxes.

"Anything else?"

"No."

"Just write the order for me, O.K.? Then go and get you something to eat."

"O.K." I pulled the green plastic folder of the University Hospital chart. The orders were ones I had written many times, a few simple lines. Yet I took an inordinate amount of time. I was procrastinating. Though, I knew most of the nurses who worked the day shift on 3-East, I felt awkward going to the luncheon.

When finished, the orders had not taken long enough.

A slender nurse with dark brown, almost black hair exited the conference room. She smiled at me as I stood indecisively, reached under the sink and returned to the party. I needed to wash my hands. As I dropped the paper towel, I realized that there was nothing left to do but enter the party. I did.

A few people spoke to me as I entered. My awkwardness began to ease. A sumptuous feast was spread across the room. I headed for the sodas. I was making small talk in the corner when Cheryl arrived.

"Dr. Saunders, how come you're not eating something? . . . Here, let me fix you a plate." She heaped mounds of food. I wondered if a paper plate could withstand Cheryl's generosity. "Here, you have some of this rice. I made it." She said proudly as she handed me the straining plate.

"Good, good." I warbled between mouthfuls of food. "This rice you made is excellent, Cheryl." It was. It really was.

"Well, thank you." Cheryl smiled inside and well as outside. She seemed finally satisfied that she had saved me from the throes of starvation, at least for one day. She left me on my own for a time.
The meal and the company were enjoyable. I grew closer to the staff of the unit during this the first of many parties given while I was on 3-East.

I led two different lives while on Urology. One, with the white coats, was as uninteresting and sterile as the urine of a normal bladder. The other was filled with the camaraderie of the staff of 3 East, people who cared for and respected one another.

CHAPTER 21

Urology often involves more psychology than physiology.

--a priest of the yellow shoes.

Three twenty-three P.M. Urology clinic was just about over. I leaned against the counter where the charts of patients who had just been seen were kept. Clinic was light and the day uncharacteristically muggy. I ambled toward the radiology conference room behind the clinic. Ed and the other house staff were seeing their last patients. The smallness of the room along with its dark red carpeting gave it a coziness and warmth that few rooms in the hospital attained. No windows opened to the outside. The quietness was relaxing and lent itself to pleasant day dreaming or, if one was not careful, sleep. I liked the room. I settled into one of the seven identical office chairs with rollers in the front row, near the view box. Dr. Gilbert, the uro-radiologist, could be heard in the next room, his office. I thought better of my position within the room as I recalled the incident with Rich Picard. With a single push of my legs, I was in the rear of the room. William Gilbert entered the conference room.

"Hi!" He said cheerily.

"Hi." I tried to sound cheerful. "How're you doing?" I asked, trying more enthusiasm than I felt.

"O.K." He smiled. "And you?"

"O.K." I said, still not able to muster much enthusiasm.

He had a way of looking at one as he spoke that made one realize that he was actually talking to one, not simply performing a social obligation.

"How're things going with you?" He looked into my eyes which I was fighting to keep open.

"O.K." I answered non-committedly. Despite his apparent openness and honesty, I was wary.

"You look tired." The priest said.

I felt bored out of my head and no small amount useless. I liked neither feeling.

"No, not really." I would not have admitted being either tired or bored for such an admission would have been a sacrilege against the God of the Knife. Bill Gilbert smiled a knowing smile. "You learning anything?"

I considered the question. After a week on Urology, it was the first time that I had done so. I had learned very little. That bothered me. "A little, I guess." I answered finally.

"That's a shame. I haven't been able to spend the time with you I would like to." The priest watched me for a second more. "I have to go downstairs now. If they want me, that's where I'll be." He left.

"O.K." I called after him.

The machine made a noise like an armored tank as Ed stepped on the petal. I sat impassively as it raced past numerous x-rays. A long stretch where no films appeared on the board was broken by the passage of two films.

"Did we just pass him there?" the chief resident asked.

Fred spoke. “I don't think so."

"What number we at now?"

"Thirty-seven."

"We must've passed it."

"No, we didn't get to it yet.

"We going forwards or backwards?"

"Backwards."

Ed pressed a second pedal. "I think we passed it." The cassette came to rest again. The chief resident pulled one of the films. He read the name aloud disgustedly. "Lester
Williams."

"See, I told you, Ed." Fred whined.

"Alright, alright." Impatience filled Ed's voice. Fred fingered a dark brown mustache which stood below a receding hair line. The number thirty-five appeared. The cassette stopped. The room was quiet as the house staff studied the films. Ed stood in front of the board, obscuring the view of everyone except Fred who stood next to him. "ED--mind if I look, too?" Matt nudged Ed out of his line of vision. "There's nothing on there, anyway." Ed's voice rose in pitch. He watched as Matt leaned forward inspecting the x-rays.

Matt sat back. "O.K."

Ed looked at his cards again. "The next one is Martinez. She on the board?"

"No, she's not on the log sheet."

"What about Myers?"

"Not here either."

Ed began looking through one of several stacks of x-ray folders. Fred and Chuck did likewise.

"Here's Myers," Fred called out.

"Is it Elena Martinez you're looking for?"

"Yeah."

"Here it is then." Munger called out. Ed threw the large pieces of plastic in front of the florescent lights. A moment of silence ensued as the priests studied the x-rays. Bone shown in gleaming white. Overlying the bone was a subtle mesh of shadows, a mystifying assortment of grays both light and dark which to the trained eye could represent rampant, uncontrolled disease or one of the myriads of patterns of normal. Using the technique gained from a renowned radiology teaching text, I began with the boney structures. Even these I found difficult to interpret because of the super-imposed gas shadows formed by the gut. I had only evaluated half the bones of the spine when, as usual, the films were removed. I was used to this. If there were any interesting findings, I would pull it later and review it with one of the radiology attendings or residents.

"See anything?" Ed asked no one in particular.

"No." Fred answered.

The chief resident pulled the film. "Let's look at Myers." As Fred mounted the films, Ed reviewed his index card on the patient.

"This is the guy with CA of the prostate, isn't it?" Fred asked. The florescent light reflecting from his glasses seemed to emanate from his eyes, giving him the appearance of an only slightly mad scientist.

"Yeah."

I hurried through my checklist again as the priests looked at the x-ray. I glanced only briefly at the bones, hoping to at least get a quick look at the outline of the kidneys and ureters. Matt leaned forward to view the films more closely.

"Alright, George, what do you see here." It was the first time that the chief resident had spoken to me during x-ray rounds. I was pleased.

However, the films were to me a befuddling conglomeration of light and dark places which appeared no more and no less than other x-rays of this type which were pronounced normal.

I knew that normal was not the correct answer. What the answer *was* not obvious to me. The priests stirred. I went through the radiology incantation as taught by a British priest. Boney structures first. They seemed all right. The psoas shadows. Difficult to make out, but normal. The renal outlines seemed normal as well. Munger cleared his throat. I rushed through the obvious renal lesions which might produce an easily identifiable x-ray abnormality. None were evident.

Impatience hung like the sword of Damocles--growing heavier as each second passed--suspended by an increasingly worn thread.

"Look at the x-ray!" Ed turned toward me while gesticulating at the florescent tubes, excitedly.

"It's really not hard." Fred called out kindly.

I glanced quickly at the gas shadows. These I knew I could quickly identify from Surgery E. The room writhed with tension. I retreated to the last defense of the ignorant—I stalled. Maybe I might pick up a needed clue with a little time.

The bones I was safe in. Even a novice priest-cadet could not go far wrong there. "The intervertebral spaces are well maintained." Munger shifted uncomfortably. "And the boney structures show some chronic arthritic changes in L- . . ." I was beginning to really get into this, sounding like a radiologist, ". . . Let me see. L 4,5'

"How could you miss that? It's so obvious." Ed nearly shouted at me. He was beginning to sweat with excitement.

"The answer is right there in front of you."

I regarded Ed's shiny face, then the view box. No answer was forthcoming.

"You've been here over a week now." Ed began a very demeaning tone. "We've gone over this again and again. What does this guy have?" Ed's voice reeked of sarcasm.

"Prostatic CA." I answered. The man had cancer of the prostate.

"What goes along with prostatic CA?"

I volunteered the only answer I knew. "Blastic lesions."

"Do you see any blastic lesions?"

Though I had not considered the association of blastic lesions and this man's diagnosis, I had looked for blastic lesions already and found none.

Again, I scrutinized the films closely. I could distinguish only the normal light and dark shadows of the overlying bowel gas. I had read about and seen examples of the densely white irregular-appearing metastases of prostatic cancer. I had yet to actually see an x-ray of such a patient except in a book. The x-ray before me resembled none I had seen in Lucy Squire's textbook. It looked depressingly normal.

"No." I answered Ed's question, indicating that I saw no blastic lesions.

The chief resident jumped from his seat as if catapulted. "What do you mean you don't see blastic lesions?" he screamed. His face turned a deep shade of pink. "They're all over the place. There and there and there . . .".

He pointed to several areas in such rapid succession that I could not pinpoint a single spot he indicated.

"You should know this." He turned to allow me the full force of his attack. "We've been over this again and again."

The warm tingling feeling of anger filled my pores and could only escape through my lips. "No one here has ever reviewed *any* x-rays with me." My lips hung on the word "any" allowing my anger to propel it across the room into the face of the chief resident. There was a tense moment of silence while I glared at the resident priest. I waited for him to say more.

He turned and sat down. The small priest with the thinning brown hair ignored the gauntlet thrown before him by one impetuous new initiate of the sacred rites. He clung helplessly, futilely to an evanescent facade of power which vanished before us even as his receding hair line.

CHAPTER 22

"The operating room is perhaps the last strong hold where the power of the priest remains unchallenged. When that goes . . ."

--a priest of the God of the Knife.

The light was soft on the yellow walls of the office we used as a lounge between cases. I had come there mainly to be out of the way as the technician moved the still sleeping patient. Other members of the Plastic Surgery Service were in various parts of the out-patient operating room, preparing for the next case. I pulled strands of unused chromic suture from my breast pocket. My legs, too long for the scrub suit when I was standing, protruded further as I sat. Threading the brittle sutures through my shoe laces, I began practicing the slickest knot I had ever seen. It had been taught to me two weeks before by Bob Sanchez, another third year student. The knot itself was nothing more than a simple square knot. The magic lay in the way it came about. The fingers of one hand weaved an intricate web while the other hand did little more than hold a single thread taunt. The truly dexterous surgeon (I was surprised to find how many possessed less dexterity than I) would perform this knot so quickly, with such ease and fluidity of motion that one was forced to let escape an involuntary "A-a-ahh".

Someone entered the room, paused a second, left. I did not look up. It would be carefully orchestrated. Between two major cases, when the entire plastic surgery team was present, I would sit down casually, paying no attention to anyone, extract a package of silk suture from my pocket (silk tied so much easier than chromic) and begin tying my one-handed knot with flowing, consummate skill.

"That boy has good hands" The voice of Isaac Kodama, plastic surgery chief resident, awoke me. He was not supposed to be there. Hours of careful plotting were wasted. Utter surprise and the realization that Isaac had been watching me for several minutes rendered my train of thought non-functional for the space of a few seconds. Kodama was a much respected and gifted operator. A wide smile of satisfaction and admiration spread across his face. I smiled back at the chief resident as I continued to tie the knot.

"Thank you." I told him.

CHAPTER 23

May our hands move with skill and swiftness as we work in the service of our God.

--prayer of the priests of the God of Surgery

The patient was a little girl. I knew nothing of the case. It, like everything else about the University Hospital, had managed to escape me over the long holiday weekend. It was the third case of the day. The others I had not known, nor did I know the case to follow.

I glanced quickly at the small figure lying on its back. The girl lay still. The anesthesiologist stood over her at the head of the table, deftly orchestrating his cluster of instruments until his efforts culminated in a breathing pattern as steady as the tread of death. He pulled the ear plug from the hole in his surgical hood. "She's ready," he announced.

The surgeons, clad in green like the anesthesiologist, moved close to look at their charge. I moved with them. "Can we put her on her stomach?" Kodama asked Zamer, the anesthesiologist.

The circulating nurse moved closer to the table.

"Yeah, but we'll need a pillow for her head." Each of us held a limb or other part of her body. The sleeping child was lifted quickly, gently, onto her abdomen. It was then that I noticed that the darkness around Sarah's neck was not due to the waist-length hair of her head. The darkness which lay over her shoulders, nearly to covering the upper part of both arms, was a furry growth. Her body suddenly took on an appearance more animal than human. I looked again at her face. It was angelic even in its death-like stillness.

Sarah was a little girl afflicted with a terrible disease. Kodama spoke to the scrub nurse. He told her which areas were to be prepared for surgery. "You better prep all the leg".

"All of it?"

"Yeah, underneath, too, so we can lift her foot up."

Kodama turned to Earl Duke, a surgical resident rotating through plastics, and me. "Let's scrub, guys."

Earl explained as we scrubbed. Sarah had what were called hairy nevi (or hairy moles) over forty percent of her body. She and a younger sib had both been born with them. Whereas his were only a few small curious patches, hers covered a substantial portion of her body. We were removing the moles for two reasons. The first was social. Earl related stories of adults who were only slightly less cruel and more tolerant than children toward Sarah. Sarah, who was beginning school and could no longer be protected by a supportive home environment, was beginning to understand the social implications of her condition. Secondly, there was a significant chance that the moles might become cancer.

As they stood above the girl's body, the surgeons' hands trembled with the holy ire of the God of the Steel Blade. My hand trembled as well, but not with excitement as I sought reason in the child's affliction.

CHAPTER 24

Surgery offers us the chance to work with patients who are essentially healthy except for their acute problem and who almost always get better after the operation. What more could you ask for?

--a resident-priest of the God of the Knife

Plastic surgery clinic. Both Kodama and Gerber were seeing patients separately.

"Hi, I'm Dr. Kodama." Isaac's long coat followed him into the exam room. "This is Dr. Saunders."

"Hi." The woman was attractive, in her mid-twenties. She hesitated for the space of a few seconds then quickly warmed.

"I . . . I had a breast operation about six months ago."

"Implants."

"Yes, that's what they call them." This woman, with skin tanned almost as deeply as her burnished brown hair, began to speak with Kodama as if he were an old friend rather than a doctor she had never seen ten minutes before. "You see, now my breasts are hard. They're not soft," she touched her chest to emphasize her point, "like they used to be." I did not fully comprehend what the woman was saying.

"Un-huh. Do they hurt?" The chief resident asked.

"No."

"Uh-huh. What happened is that the body sometimes has a reaction to the material and forms a hard substance around the implant."

"Does that mean I'm allergic to them?" Her face was concern.

"No, no." Kodama smiled reassuringly. "It just means that there are some fibrous areas which need to be broken down." He turned to me. "You see what happens sometimes is that cysts form with fibrous bands around the implant. They can make the breasts very hard."

"I *see."* I said

"Once you break down the cysts, the breasts become soft again."

The woman interrupted Kodama. "What do you mean 'break down the cysts?'" She looked worried.

"We-e-ell," Kodama turned to the woman, "What we do is apply pressure until they pop. In other words, we squeeze them real hard."

The woman looked more worried. "Does that hurt?"

"Well, we give you something so that you don't feel it very much."

"Do I have to come back for that or do you do it now?"

"We'll do it now."

"0h . . . O.K."

Kodama opened the door wide enough to stick his head through. "Cynthia?" he yelled. Someone in another room answered. "Ten milligrams Valium I.V., please!"

We waited half a minute.

"Where's the Valium?"

"Just a minute, just a minute." Cynthia chided gently as she glided into the room. "Here it is." She held a small syringe of clear yellow fluid.

"This 10 milligrams?"

"Ye-es." She teased the chief resident.

Silently, very interested I watched as Kodama slowly pushed in half the contents of the syringe.

"How do you feel?"

"O.K." her voice was tremulous.

Kodama waited a few seconds. "Feel sleepy yet?"

"No." her voice wavered less. "Just kind of . . . "

"Woozy?" Kodama asked. "Feel like you're going to pass out?" He watched her face.

"No, just kind of tingly."

He pushed the remainder of the yellow fluid into her arm. Fifteen seconds passed.

"Well, how do you feel now?"

"Kind of relaxed. You know kind of . . . "

"O.K." Kodama's manner was all business. "You're going to feel some discomfort now for just a second. O.K.?"

"O.K."

Isaac quickly separated the opening of the woman's gown. He placed the entire breast between his two palms. I noticed for the first time that though the chief resident was short he was powerfully built.

"Ready?" Before the woman could answer he pushed the heels of his palms together. A horrible, gut-busting, crackling pop was heard half a second before the woman's scream. I grimaced involuntarily barely managing not to cry out, myself. Tears flooded the woman's face. Kodama's expression was one of smug satisfaction.

"That hurt!" She sniffled. "Oh, that hurt."

"It's all over now, dear." Isaac tone was paternal. "You go ahead and get dressed now." Isaac left the room.

"If I knew it was going to hurt this much, I wouldn't have had it done. They should give you some kind of anesthesia or something." The young woman whimpered. She blew her nose as I closed the door behind me.

Several patients still waited. I followed the long coat into the room.

"Hi. I'm Dr. Gerber." The attending priest was short with thinning, walnut colored hair which he wore long and combed over a bare patch of scalp. "This is a medical student working in the clinic." He indicated me. "He doesn't have to be here if you don't want him to."

"No, that's quite alright." She spoke calmly, not bothered. She was a very pretty, well-built woman, whom I judged to be somewhere in her thirties. Her smooth brown skin was of the variety ever imbued with youth. I recognized her face from the V.A. hospital where I had exchanged greetings with her several times.

"If you don't want to discuss this in front of him, he can wait outside, you know." Enough already! I began to wonder if the attending priest was uncomfortable with my presence.

She answered evenly. "I don't mind if he stays." I was pleased.

"Well, what can we do for you?" he asked resignedly.

"Well, you see doctor, it's my breasts." Gerber nodded.

"Look at me. I'm thirty-four but my body is that of a twenty-five year old. I haven't gained a pound since I was in high school. I eat right. I exercise. I do lots of good things to stay in shape. I really do. People always compliment me on my figure, how nice it is. But these breasts, doctor--they don't look like they belong to the same body."

Unlike with the previous patient I had seen with him, Gerber did not force the patient to elaborate with help as third year clerks were taught to do. He somehow understood what she spoke of. I did also. She was quite right. While the rest of her body was firm and shapely, her breasts hung limply before her.

"Do you want them larger, too?"

"No, I just don't want them to hang like this."

"O.K., we'll schedule you for surgery in a month."

"Can't I have it sooner?"

"We can't schedule you before that. We're booked up already."

"Well, O.K." she said reluctantly. She did not know that she was having her surgery at a very early date. The usual wait was anywhere from six to twelve weeks. This was done purposely to allow those who might change their mind ample time to do so.

Gerber passed into the corridor. I paused at the doorway. "Bye." I smiled gratefully.

"Bye."

During the rest of the day I kept coming back to the ease with which this woman discussed the most intimate details of her life with two strangers. This power of the priesthood was one which still awed me years afterward.

CHAPTER 25

Let Courage be our constant companion as we follow the path of our God.

--prayer of the student-priests

Consult rounds. I followed the long white coat of Kodama, closely.

"You're going to the V.A. hospital." Isaac told me. I groaned. Plastic surgery at the V.A. meant skin flaps, skin flaps, skin flaps. Boring! The major portion of the plastic surgery at the V.A. would be devoted to covering bed sores.

Maybe it was only for a day or better yet a special lecture. Yeah, maybe a lecture.

Isaac spoke. "Maybe a week or so."

"A week?"

"How much longer you here with us anyway?" Isaac did not respond to the disappointment in my voice.

"About ten days."

"Ten days, huh? You might finish up out there. They're getting pretty busy out there. They could use some help, especially since things have kind of slacked off here."

Though I liked the V.A. more than the U., I did not want to do plastic surgery there.

The decision to shift the rotation around had actually come as no surprise. A few days before, I had had lunch with my counter-part at the V.A. He had stated that they were becoming over-worked as the sub-intern's rotation had ended and the case load had increased. The only other plastic surgery resident besides Kodama was thus working at the V.A. with the aid of only a third year clerk. I knew also that the lack of variety seen at the V.A. concerned the faculty.

They wanted both students on the rotation to see as many types of cases as possible. I had thought however that they might bring the other student down for part of the week. I empathized with my colleague, but I did not want to join him.

□ □ □ □

Lunchtime. The U. I stood behind Kodama in line. Would it be the entrees which I knew I could not afford or the usual over-cooked and dry hamburger?

"He-e-ey, Damian! What's up?" Isaac spoke to a slender long coat with dark hair and mustache. He was younger than Isaac.

"Hi, Isaac!" They began an animated conversation. While they spoke, I read the name tag. Damian White. He was the other chief resident in plastic surgery. Somehow, he seemed too young, too fresh scrubbed for the job. He did not compare to Isaac. More than the few years, perhaps two or three, difference in their ages. Kodama, the shorter of the two, towered over White. Also, Kodama's manner with White was not that of an equal but rather that of one speaking to someone a step below him. I later found that Kodama had survived the University's vicious pyramid system and was board certified in general surgery. He was then completing his second of two years in plastic surgery. White had come upon his position in plastic surgery after only three years in a general surgery program. As an afterthought, Isaac introduced us. "This is George Saunders. He'll probably come up and help you guys out."

"George, this is Damian White." I extended my hand and smiled politely. There seemed an unwarranted coldness in the man as he extended a purely perfunctory limp fish. I shook it. He spoke to Isaac. "We're doing O.K., Isaac. We don't need any help."

A week later. I was still at the U.

□ □ □ □

Water, tinged brown from betadine, dripped from my hands. I entered the room buttocks first, carefully following the cleansing ritual which had become second nature to me. I also adhered strictly to the rules of surgical etiquette which demanded that I, the lowest member of the team, enter last. I waited patiently as the green clothed and masked figures of Kodama, Gerber, and White prepared the subject sacrifice to the God of Learning, a God whose eyes faced in every direction and whose hundred arms and thousand fingers explored, touched, probed all they came near. I waited patiently, as I was ignored.

The waiting held no animosity for my presence was often helpful and served to the benefit of the patient. My waiting was necessitated by expediency. I was fascinated by the battle of blood and gore in which the surgeons began with a wrongful, diseased order, made chaos, then made an order all their own. I enjoyed witnessing, being a part of the working of the priests' magic.

While the patient was being draped and the major actors of the drama, the attending and chief resident priest still needed her assistance, Wilke, the scrub nurse tossed a towel onto my still wet hands. I smiled and said thank you loudly, perhaps too loudly. She looked at me as if remembering a resident or an attending whom she had helped thusly and who now thought himself too powerful and important to give her the time of day. I neither forgot her courtesy, nor that of other nurses who first taught me to draw blood, to start an I.V., to write orders, or who taught me any of a thousand other secrets of the priesthood.

“Towel clips." Gerber called the scrub nurse back to the table.

"They're right at your fingertips, doctor." She returned her attention to the priest.

"Can I have the marking solution?" A small sterilized glass bowl containing a blue inky material was placed on the patient’s bare chest. Two over-large mounds of flesh which would have blended into near anonymity if not for their enormous size protruded from the woman's chest.

Carefully, with surprising artistry, Gerber drew concentric circles and bands like the illustrations of a geometric three-dimensional figure. His strokes were fluid motion. Lines were laid out deftly, connected, with no signs of hesitancy or ambiguity. A second stolen moment and my gown was on. Wilke held the chord, while I twirled quickly, completing my cleansing ritual. She handed the chord of my gown back to me. I thanked her.

Gerber handed the marking solution to White. I moved to the side of the patient where Kodama and Gerber stood. Etiquette demanded that I stand on the opposite side with Damian. I feigned ignorance. I had heard about White in the O.R. His reputation was that of a hog who hoarded even the minor tasks for himself and gave nothing but blame to his assistants. I hoped that Gerber might scrub out or simply observe while Kodama operated. I might get a chance to assist or at the very least I could watch unbothered.

White began to draw the lines of the battle plan to reduce the breasts too large for even this over-large framed woman, breasts which caused her almost constant pain. The resident priest was not bad. His lines, however, were not as smooth as those of the attending physician, nor did they match those of the opposite size. Gerber took the ink-filled bowl.

"We want to make them both even, Damian." Gerber dipped the wooden stick which served as a pen in the solution.

"This line should go more like this." He redrew the line so that it matched that on the opposite side. "There." He passed the bowl off the operating field.

The pace of the operation was more leisurely than Kodama's usual brisk pace. Gerber was in charge. Kodama remained silent except to ask for tools to assist the attending priest. Gerber intended to operate. Carefully the knife blade bisected the marks he had made.

"You want me to begin on this side?" White directed his question to the attending.

Gerber looked up. "Sure, why don't you start."

"Skin knife." Wilke passed the scalpel to Damian.

"George?" The attending priest addressed me.

"Yes?" I almost stood at attention.

"You go on that side and assist Damian." I swore silently. I moved without hesitation, without uttering a word. Gerber was low key, but still a surgeon. Once on the other side of the patient, I placed my hands on the familiar and safe neutral green of the abdomen. For the space of a few seconds I observed White. He was still making the skin incision. I placed my hands on both sides of the incision, careful not to obstruct his view and applied pressure as was customary.

"Don't do that! I'll tell you when I what I want you to do."

I removed my hands, placing them both on the neutral green of the abdomen. A moment later, when the formless, moving mass became unmanageable, he spoke to me. "Here. Put your hand here." He indicated the same spot where my hand had been before. "Just use one hand. I'll get the other side." I complied, saying nothing. I took note of the time. It was going to be a long operation. Kodama and Gerber continued without problems. Damian followed their progress. Small bleeding vessels, called "bleeders", appeared frequently. Damian worked feverishly clamping the vessels. The next step was to cauterize the bleeders. I held the clamp to expedite the process as Kodama did for Gerber and as I had done countless times before.

"Don't touch that!" Damian snapped. Kodama and Gerber looked up briefly, said nothing, then returned to their work.

White continued. A thin squirting stream of blood left the table hitting me in the chest, then the face. White tried twice to clamp it unsuccessfully. I sponged once quickly to clear the field and aid his search.

"Don't do that." The resident snapped. "Now, I can't find it."

"What's the matter, Damian? You got a bleeder over there?"

"Yeah."

"Damian, we're getting wet over here." Gerber joked.

"Yeah, look at George." Kodama chuckled.

White searched for the vessel again. I could see it well with my right eye only as the left lens of my glasses was splattered with blood. Each heart beat sprayed more of the red liquid in my face. The

metallic click of the hemostat sounded as the resident missed a third time. A small hemostat lay on the table in front of me. Annoyance finally overcame me. I grabbed the instrument and with one deft move
clamped the bleeder. I looked pointedly, stone-faced, at the far wall. Neither my action nor my expression were lost on Gerber or Kodama. They looked at my splattered glasses, my gown, at Damian. They proceeded with the operation, allowing thinly disguised mirth to play across their faces.

"Told you not to do anything until . . . "

"Yeah!" I cut him off. My expression did not change. Damian said little else during the remainder of the procedure. I was glad.

Surgery completed. We removed our gowns at the sink. "Boy look like you took a bath in it." We all laughed.

"Somebody ought to get a picture of you." As I stood before the mirror, I could only agree that I was quite a gruesome sight.

Later I recounted to my classmates the tale of the thrice missed vessel and my valorous conclusion to the problem. They laughed heartily. Tales of a coup by a medical student were always well received.

CHAPTER 26

Virtually all cures in medicine belong to the realm of surgery. All other medical specialties are concerned largely with the palliation of chronic disease.

--lectures of the priests of the God of the knife

The sedate quietness did not dispel the subdued terror. I was one of the last to be called. My colleagues talked in subdued tones of the coming trial. A few asked questions. The answers they knew, but feigned ignorance. I had long ago seen through this deception. I pointedly ignored them. They left me alone. The real test, a three-part oral exam for surgery was approaching quickly--too quickly.

Dausman leafed feverishly through a surgical book, a pocket-sized tome in a popular science and medical series. I liked the series on medicine. It was clear, concise with excellent references. It was the kind of book you could read in fifteen minutes if you knew you were going be quizzed on a given topic. But time was too short and the subject too broad.

"How am I going to know all this stuff?" Ernie chewed his nails as he spoke. I wondered was it possible to live on a diet of nails as Ernie seemed to do when he was uptight about something. He swore under his breath.

"Ernie, why don't you put the book away?" I spoke though I preferred silence. I found it hard to watch Dausman torment himself.

"Ernest Dausman." A long-coated priest called out. Ernie looked up.

"You'll do O.K." I tried not to let my own trepidation show in my voice.

A voice sounded. A second priest also wearing a long coat called my name. Both Ernie and I rose. Two priest-cadets smiled the secret smile of the sacrificial lamb as they approached the alter of the God of the Knife.

I followed the priest into his office. He slumped into a large chair behind his desk. Tiredness was a heavy weight pulling at the edges of the priest's face. I remained standing, awaiting an invitation to be seated.

"Go ahead, sit down," the priest told me. He was one of the younger faculty. His hair was a deep brown.

I sat quickly, quietly, rigidly.

The priest spoke my name. "I'm going to give you some questions and I want you to answer them." I felt sorry for the priest. He was obviously exhausted. Mine was perhaps his fourth or fifth exam of the afternoon. He grasped several sheets of neatly typed paper. He read from these the first of several scenarios. The history was that of a person with gastro-intestinal bleeding. From Surgery E, I could handle G.I. bleeders in my sleep. I calmly ran through a plan of initial treatment along with the appropriate tests and procedures. Every so often he would place the paper back on the desk to make a mark. He was evidently marking off a checklist as I made the required points. I continued with my list of differential diagnoses. He stopped me.

"That's fine, that's fine." He looked at the paper then at me.

"Let's go on to the next one." He was impressed. We went through several more questions, a total of approximately twelve. I answered all but two completely. Even these I answered partially.

The priest looked at his watch. "We're finished early." He smiled at me gratefully. "Maybe the next student might be out, then we can get out of here early."

"Well, thank you." I smiled as I rose.

"Bye now."

"Bye." I walked into the outer waiting area.

I sat only a moment before my name was called again. As I followed the second interviewer to his office, my eyes rested upon the glistening circle of pale pink skin encompassed by a thin band of closely cropped hair. I was impressed that Locke was brilliant, strait-laced, and aloof. His immaculate white coat remained stiffly at his side as he walked as if ordered to attention. His manner was polite, but bothered. He did not enjoy this process. I answered each of the questions he asked. Unlike the first examiner, he was difficult to read. I felt that I acquitted myself well, though. I was quite pleased thus far. I had answered the questions put to me far beyond the depth required by my examiners. All my hours of toil, of poring over charts, staying beyond the required time, of pestering house staff with questions had paid off. Still, however, there was the third examiner. Pessimistically, I speculated that lurking somewhere in one of the offices of the complex, was a priest sent directly by the sanguine God of the Knife to humiliate me and drive away nascent courage. I waited uneasily for my third interview. Perhaps the God of the Knife might yet show mercy on this fledgling initiate to the rites of the priesthood. The talking in the waiting area among the students who remained reached an audible roar. Locke called another name. The student followed him with a fearful gait that was uncomfortable pained and familiar. I listened intently to the conversation of two of my colleagues. Dausman was not out yet. I hoped he was doing well. The dialogue between my classmates was animated and worried.

"George, you want to come with me." I was startled. I had not seen the tall broad-shouldered priest approach. Above me stood the surgery core course director. I had seen him many times, but had never had the opportunity or need to speak with him directly. I was surprised, though I should not have been, that he spoke my name as if it were one very familiar to him. This same thing happened frequently during medical school. Instructor often knew my name before our first meeting.

"Down this way." I rose and followed the priest. He closed the door behind me. "Sit down, George." He motioned to a chair in front of his desk.

"Thank you."

He sat down. "You holding up under all the questions so far?" He smiled.

"So far, O.K."

"Good." He looked down at a sheet of paper. "I have a few more for you." He began questions on fluid and electrolytes. The topic was one which confounded many attending physicians. I made pretense of nothing but the most rudimentary knowledge of the subject. My confidence evaporated. Still, I answered all the questions in short
order. There were fewer questions than with the previous interviewers. I wondered why?

My examiner leaned back in his chair, poising a pencil in his fingertips. "How did you like the rotation?" So that was it. This was the place where they obtained feedback from the students. I knew better than to answer a question like that one without knowing exactly what my interviewer wanted to hear.

"How do you mean?" I asked, watching his face warily.

"Do you think you learned anything?"

"Yes, a great deal." It was true.

"What about the surgical sub-specialties? Some people thought that three weeks was too long."

"Really?" I asked the priest.

"Yes, some students thought particularly on electives like Urology and Neuro-surgery that three weeks was too long."

"I know particularly on rotations like plastic surgery that there were many skills I acquired which I would not have been able to in a two-week rotation."

He seemed thoughtful. "Yes, that's true." He pondered. "I know that some of the students had some problems on

Urology." So, he knew about Rich Picard and Ed Rind. "How did you find it?"

"No problems." I said straight faced. I did not mention the time I was set to strangle Ed. I was probably the only student who did not complain about the chief resident of Urology. We chatted for a few more minutes, then I took my leave. I was impressed that the course director was a sincere man. I liked him.

Rumor had it that he was leaving the University because of his conflicts with the chair of the department. I hoped that the rumors were not true. If they were, there would be a great loss to both the Department and the University.

CHAPTER 27

To evade an unpleasant truth is to give it more importance than it deserves.
--the Heretic Priest

The summer dwindled into its final days of lazy warmth. Dressed in comfortable jeans, a navy-blue T-shirt which was embroidered with a multicolored coastal scene, and a slightly stretched denim jacket, I made my way slowly over the vine covered hillock. I avoided the wooden steps which antedated the University and which had reached a dangerous state of disrepair as I traversed the several hundred yards from the V.A. hospital to the University campus proper. A few ground squirrels stopped their foraging as I approached, eyed me suspiciously, then vanished in a small cloud of dust. The shuttle made its way by a rather circuitous route, the only route for vehicles, to the medical school campus. Sometimes I liked the long, lonely walk from the V.A. to the offices of the campus. It gave me time to think. Often when I was required to make this long trek, I needed the time to prepare myself for the sometimes-unpleasant tasks which brought me to the medical school. This day, however, the tasks were not unpleasant. I was there to see my surgery evaluations and make a social call at the Minority Recruitment Office. As I approached, I could see a young woman dressed in baggy jeans, and a loose-fitting sweat shirt. Martha

Livingston, the director of the MRO, spoke to the woman. Martha wore many hats. She worked with the undergraduate students as well as those in the school of medicine. Her office was one of a coveted few in the new medical school administrative complex. I smiled when I thought how it had come about. Two years before, Martha's office had existed on paper only. The building in which it had been housed had been demolished with no plans for moving the MRO. We students had deftly put together a multiracial front of both students and faculty which went before the dean of the medical school to put forth some pragmatic solutions to the problem. The end result was the office I approached. I was quite proud of both the political acumen of the students and the office. Martha did a lot of good things for a lot of people, making her value to the school go far beyond the confines of her title. The door to the office of student affairs (OSA) opened. A very young appearing, casually dressed man with chestnut colored hair falling over the edges of his ears, exited. As I caught the metal door, I wondered had I looked so young, freshly scrubbed and untried as this young man, some three years before when I had entered medical school. I hoped I had not. Uneasiness settled upon me quickly, easily as the door closed behind me. I looked into several smiling faces. The bright new office, the sunshine, and a new dean of student affairs could not erase the plethora of bad memories associated with the OSA. I returned a smile which I hoped was not as superficial as the feeling within it or as I thought those showed me. I looked for the single face, brown like my own, which I had lately begun to trust. Trudy was not there.

"Can I help you with something, George?" one of the clerks offered.

"Yes, I heard that the surgery evaluations are in." "Yes. You want yours?"

"Yes, thank you."

"I'll get them for you." A very pale black-haired woman rose. I leaned against the counter as she disappeared into a back office. The door opened. Another third year student stood next to me.

"Hi, Dan." I spoke to my colleague. The student-priest was somewhat of a celebrity because he lived with a woman in the first-year class. They were a frequent topic of medical school gossip.

"Hi, George." he answered in a mildly solicitous tone which was his normal way of talking.

"What're you doing?" He smiled.

"Oh, looking at my surgery evaluations."

"Yeah, the one's from medicine aren't done yet."

"You took medicine first?" I asked.

"Yeah."

"You got a bad draw. huh?" I referred to the lottery which determined the order in which each student took clerkships.

"No, I just wanted to get it out of the way."

"Boy!" I looked at him incredulously. I did not believe that any sane person would voluntarily take medicine, the clerkship most feared by students, without a little ward experience first. "You're brave." He chuckled at my comment.

"What're you doing here?" I asked. I did not hear his answer because my attention was drawn to the plain manila folder which the woman held in her hands.

"We can't let these out. You'll have to look at it here. Let's see, . . . " She looked thoughtfully about the room. "Why don't you look at them in here?" She indicated a small bare room with a desk. "Barbara is not using her office."

"Excuse me." I called to Dan.

"Take it easy."

As I approached the room where she stood, she placed the folder on the desk. She smiled as she passed. "Let me know when you're done." I sat down. It took me a few minutes to figure out the grading system. It was not simply the narrative style I had been used to for the first two years of medical school. It was divided into about two dozen characteristics, each of which was followed by four columns which the evaluator was to check. The labels to the column--outstanding, excellent, adequate, fair—were remarkably like the A, B, C, D system I was used to as an undergraduate. I studied the unfamiliar array of marks. The categories of evaluation included everything from personal appearance to relationships with house staff to cognitive knowledge. There were several checks in the excellent column, a host of them under adequate, and a few in the fair column. I was crushed.

I looked at the narrative comments. No comment at all was made about the many, many hours of extra work I had put in on the wards. I deserved better, much, much better. I swore under my breath. I fought to control the anger deep within me, anger augmented by an overwhelming sense of betrayal. It was not the first time I had been left with this feeling, nor would it be the last. The metal door opened. Trudy returned from lunch. I steeled myself for my exit. Many times, I had seen, or imagined that I had seen, silent gloating in the eyes of the OSA staff as I had left the dean's office after one of many personal setbacks, but there had never been any acquiescence in my eyes or my bearing. I would leave the office the same way I entered—proud. Trudy watched me as I carried the manila folder. She
said nothing. I found it difficult not to acknowledge her presence.

"Hi." I said stiffly, looking toward but not at her.

"Hi." She answered, watching me closely.

"You finish with that now?" The woman who had given me the file smiled as she spoke.

"Yes, thank you." I answered, again stiffly. I opened the door and walked through it.

Martha was in the passageway. I was headed back to the V.A.

"You're not going to stop by?" Martha and I had been through many battles together. It was very rare that I passed the MRO and did not stop to say hello.

"No, I have some things to do." I tried to say calmly. She looked closely at my face. "You O.K.?" Her Missouri accent thickened.
I tried to sound reassuring as I spoke.

"Sure." She watched me silently for a second.

"Look, I really do have to go."

"O.K., then. Don't let me hold you."

"O.K., Martha, take care."

"O.K., you too."

"Bye, now."

"Bye." I walked on. (Later, after talking with my classmates, I found that mine had been one of the better evaluations. The priests of the Knife were a sanguine lot.)

I needed the long walk back to the V.A. As I retraced my steps over a lonely walkway, a tower of steel and stone made its way slowly, deliberately across a vine-covered hillock.

CHAPTER 28

She touches me
and I smile inside.
--an unsung poet

Summer was a gentle sigh carried lovingly on the wing beat of a sparrow. Summer, the season of warmth, when the orange-red sun carried on a lingering love affair with the pale azure sky. Summer, the season of unabashed warmth which reaches out to stroke the winter-laden soul. Summer, the season when the harvest reaches its opulent most. Summer, the season of overflowing fullness and abundance. Summer, the season of my birth. I was feeling a deep primeval urge to wander, to explore new vistas, to tread paths never dreamed before. The summer had been difficult, but rewarding in many ways.

I had worked slavishly through most of surgery, but I had attained a great amount of knowledge for my toil. I had lived without Grace, and for the first time had realized that we might never be together again. Also, from the hours of lonely, heart-wrenching solitude had come the realization that I could survive without her. I had fallen on my face with more than a single woman. Yet from each of these escapades, I was able to salvage the smallest kernel of self-confidence, that though vulnerably, frightened, and hurt, I could still struggle and attain some measure of success.

THE THIRD YEAR

Even the breakdown of my car and my inability to have it fixed because of lack of funds had left me with a small sum of money which usually would have been spent on routine maintenance. As the car had broken down after I had begun my rotations at the University Hospital which was a half-mile from my house, I was not greatly inconvenienced.

I felt a stirring deep within me, as ancient as that within my loins, and more urgent. I needed to leave the gold-green summer hills of Canon. I needed the open bareness away from the coast, the lush greenness of Atlantic Mexico. I needed to explore parts of Mexico which I saw only in the sunset-filled eyes of others. I needed to go quickly, deeply to a place where I was not known and where I knew no one. I needed to fill the vastness, the emptiness within me. Perhaps it was nothing more than an atavistic urge to recapture an earlier, happy time in my life when I had traveled to the shores of the Sea of Cortez and laughed care free among the gulls and warm, turquoise waves. Perhaps my thinking was escapist and unrealistic. I did not care how far I got. I knew only, in the depths of my soul, I needed
to get away.

These were my thoughts that warm summer afternoon when the tingling of the phone imparted a sense of distant urgency to the air.

It was Grace.

"Hi, honey". Her voice was melodic.

"Oh, hi. How are you doing?"

"O.K., I guess." She answered in that sweet little girl voice which always touched a special part of me. I knew something was up, but I was softened to whatever it was. I stretched out my entire length, dark and skinny across the gold softness of my bedspread. The picture of a leopard cub looked down upon me. The stretching of sinews driven into a state of dull numbness by endless hours of abuse and the almost total lack of proper exercise was good. So, too, was the slow release, the sound of gentle thunder in my ears and the ensuing yawn.

"You still there?"

"Yes. I was just stretching."

"I'm having a little problem." She paused the slightest fraction of a second. "They're going to throw me out because I'm behind in my rent."

Who were they? Throw you out of where? My mind for reasons unknown to me could not focus on these entities. A second elapsed. Throw her out of her apartment, that's what they are going to do. I was back into the here and now, but only briefly. My mind, nominally under my control, began to think of obvious, immediate solutions to Grace's problem. A solution, simple, immediate, and hurtful, raced to my consciousness. She could move in with me. The neatness, the succinct completeness of it appealed to a mind, as mine, ruled mainly by logic, but, within me, a visceral rebellion rose. Its source, not at all difficult to pinpoint, was the happenings of only a few months before when Grace had decided to move back in with me. I had been elated with the news. In the space of four hours, while she was at work, I had moved and cleaned her entire apartment. When I had arrived for the final load, I had met my bride on the doorstep, crying. What was the matter? I had asked.

"I don't want to leave here." She had answered.

"What do you mean?"

"I don't want to move back in with you." I had felt a physical pain in the space where my heart beat. It was so very real. Anger, humiliation had risen with the pain and allowed me to stay the floodgate of tears within me. A cool, logical mind had presided then also. I had suggested that she move in with me as she had already given up her apartment, until she found another. She had and had soon
left again.

The wound was too fresh. I could not suggest that she move in with me. The greater sadness was that if she asked, I could not refuse. I waited breathlessly in a sea thick with silence. Her little girl voice, the one I always loved, began again. A few seconds passed before I could focus on her words.

"Do you have any money?"

Her question registered.

"A little." Indeed, it was very little and once gone I would get no more.

"You think you could loan me enough to pay the back rent?" The little girl voice continued.

But what about the summer-gold hills of northern Mexico, the refreshing greenness of Guadalajara, the Atlantic coast? What about the other solution which I could neither live with nor refuse?

The wind played gently on the piece of paper as I signed my name.

I wrote Grace a check for three hundred dollars and a sun-imbued dream.

The price for my sanity was small.

CHAPTER 29

Empathy is an innate capacity within each of us. Our training, at times inhumane, both before and after we reach these halls, sometimes causes us to lose sight of this capacity. We can and must re-awaken, re-learn it. The rewards reach far beyond our professional lives, our relationships with our charges. Our rewards are very personal and may include sanity itself.

--the Heretic Priest

Somewhere in the male psyche is the notion that women enjoy pelvic exams. There is an unwritten and often unstated belief that some primordial urge akin to the naked unencumbered need for sexual gratification drives them to the doctor's office to have a pelvic examination. Aside from the obvious issues of sexism involved in this notion, it is difficult, I believe, for any male to comprehend the monumental complexity of the female reproductive system. Even among health professionals it takes an exceptionally sensitive individual to break through these barriers to develop compassion for the very real and often bothersome, to both patient and physician, non-specific complaints with which women frequently present. The problem, like its solutions, are not easy.

□ □ □ □

The woman was mean. There was no other way to describe her. She was just plain mean.

It was the next to last day of the two-week lecture series which preceded our release onto the pediatric and obstetrics-gynecology wards. No priests were present, only we priest-cadets having our largely male egos flailed by this small, yet somehow large woman with shoulder length brown hair. She was perhaps five feet, five inches tall, small framed, about one hundred fifteen pounds. Her pink skin had an uneven texture which looked like the aftermath of several prison riots, but which probably had no more sinister origin than severe, pitting acne. She looked us each in the eye. Each answered according to his fashion, trying to stare her down (unsuccessfully) or avoiding her gaze. I chose to look at the other women with her who
watched us with a much less menacing pose.

"We did not agree to do this job for the money they give us." We priest-cadets looked up at this. It sounded like the beginning of a confession, a small rent in the perfect armor through which we might gain access to a view of the wonder and vulnerability within. It sounded like the truthful beginning of the answer to a question we had all been asking. Why were they here? Why had these women volunteered to act as models, instructing us in how to do a pelvic exam?

What could cause them to appear before us without clothing and allow each of four strangers to place his clumsy, pain-laden fingers in her vagina? The speculations regarding this were legion. Most of them could be summed up in a few dirty jokes, a knowing smile, a smutty wink.

"All of us are professional women." There was a plaintiveness beyond the toughness, somehow more discomforting than the brusque exterior. "We are all either nurses or nurse practitioners." I shifted uncomfortably.

"We are here for one reason only." Each student-priest looked
up, even those like myself who had contented themselves with watching the designs in the floor tiles.

"We care about the health care of women." Her voice rang with sincerity. She continued. "Some of you think this is funny, that all of this is pointless, so much nonsense. Some of you think that when a woman is on that table having a pelvic exam, she gets some sort of strange sexual pleasure--well, she doesn't."

She looked around the room. The few persisting smirks began to fade rapidly.

"I've listened to a lot of woman talk about their doctors. Most of them hate to see the gynecologist. A few like going. A few, a very few, even have a crush on their doctor," A few smirks began to re-appear. " but none of them like pelvic exams!"

The lips of the student-priests were stone.

□ □ □ □ □

During the teaching of the manual skills, each group of four students was split into two groups of two. Dausman and I were together. We both felt uncomfortable about the exam and had elected to be the second of Marie's groups. We sat nervously at a round wooden table. Bob Sanchez approached. Bob, who looked the way I imagined Kahlil Gibran did, was dressed in his usual casual style. He wore green cords, a printed cotton shirt, and blue waist length ski jacket. A few students followed.

"You guys still waiting?" he asked us.

"Yeah, we're the last group." Dausman answered. "How did yours go?" he asked distractedly.

"We had Linda. She was great."

"Yeah, she just walked you straight through it." a second student added.

"Linda's a real good looker, too." Bob continued. A few smiles went around. "You know they told us about a woman not being stimulated, but they didn't tell us what to do if the doctor gets stimulated. What do you do?"

"Ask her for her phone number." Someone called out. We all laughed.

"Seriously," Bob continued. "I asked Linda."

All ears pricked up.

"You asked her for her phone number?"

"No. When I was examining her, I asked her what to do if you get an erection while examining a patient?"

"You really asked her that?"

"Sure." I believed him and was only mildly disgusted.

"What did she say?"

"She just smiled." Bob smiled also as he said this.

Conversation trickled into quietness as Ernie and I were called.

After our time of instruction, I remember leaving the building with Marie. I do not remember how this came about. Though it was not intentional, I did enjoy it.

"You know you have a very gentle touch." she looked into my face earnestly.

There was a lot to like about Marie, I thought as I watched her cinnamon eyes. I smiled. "Thank you."

"You know you should go into gynecology. You're very sensitive and would be very good at it."

My smile broadened. "Thank you again. I'll give it some thought."

"You really should."

A pleasant silence ensued for a few paces.

"What do think of the pelvic models?"

I hesitated a moment as much to gather my thoughts as to make certain that nothing hurtful came out. I liked Marie. Yes, there was a lot to like about her. She was charming, bright, warm, good-looking. Though I was attracted to her, I did not dare broach the wall of professionalism. I was too shy and afraid to venture yet another rejection. I had come to expect a rebuff from every corner.

I could see that she liked me. I chose, perhaps rightly, perhaps wrongly, to believe that this was simply the attraction of two fellow travelers basking in the joy of our shared Africaness.

Marie mistook my hesitation for not understanding her question.

She looked in my face. "Do the guys say anything to you?"

I knew the question she was really asking. What she wanted to know was if the models were thought of as fellow professionals or some kind of bimbos? The students by and large understood the reasons of the models for being there. How to tell her?

"I think we are all grateful for the experience . . ." I said, my eyes searching the sky for words. "We need . . . It's much less threatening to us . . . It's very helpful to us," I began again, striking upon the appropriate arrangement of words, "to be able to examine someone who can give honest, critical feedback regarding how we do a pelvic. You are the only ones who will do that. Also, I know that I would not have felt half the things I did if not for you."

Marie smiled warmly. We walked a few more paces, then said goodbye. Gladness and goodness were mixed with various shades of brown and black as a red-gold sun left the western sky.

CHAPTER 30

The Child God is a happy God.
--Priests of the God of Children

The pace of life was quite different on pediatrics. There were so many doctors and so few patients that the interns did not pretend to need the assistance of the students. In fact, after a short period, the interns began giving us small tasks to accomplish simply to get us out of their hair.

The prevailing attitude of the surgeons toward medical students was one of acceptance if only to perform the menial tasks, commonly called "scut," of patient care. We were to be used to hold retractors, as messengers, as blood drawers, as whipping posts to indulge the foul moods of house staff, as the butt of jokes in which gross ignorance bordered on slapstick humor, and as the sacrificial lamb to the God of the Blade when Infection and Hemorrhage had done their mischief.

Through it all we were needed. More than this, there was an esprit de corps which was not quite like that found in any other medical specialty. This feeling of camaraderie was felt by all and was the final precept which governed the actions of each member of the team. Despite the back biting, insults, and abuse, all were part of the family and treated as such.

Pediatrics, likewise had its camaraderie, somewhat more diffuse, and certainly less strong. It ended, however, with the interns. The medical students were looked upon as usurpers, perpetrators of unwarranted invasions on the unprotected bodies of children. We were tolerated, but kept always on a short leash. I resented this more than, my three colleagues who, like me, had just finished surgery and were quite happy with the much less demanding pace of pediatrics. Though boredom continued unabated, my resentment at being a purposeless cog in an interminably slow machine was soon quelled as my personal life settled into a pattern of less turmoil. The quiet times now were not always filled with longing for Grace. I began to enjoy hours away from the hospital in which I indulged in an unstructured search for fulfillment and serenity within myself.

CHAPTER 31

In the struggle against disease we must decide which battles we can win, which we cannot, and which are not worth fighting.
--Academy lectures

Morning. Work rounds. Pediatrics. She was a pretty, blond haired little girl, three or four years of age. The students had only been involved peripherally with the patient. She was the victim of a near-drowning in the family swimming pool. The peds residents, interns, and attending had worked feverishly throughout the night to save whatever brain function she might have left. We students knew without being told that this case was one we could not touch. We satisfied ourselves with glimpses gleaned from a craning neck as the Pediatric Intensive Care Unit door opened to admit one consultant or another.

Cold water drownings were discussed at length as there had been several documented cases of return to normal brain function after more than twenty minutes of submersion. Most of these reports had come from Scandinavia where it was postulated that the extremely cold-water temperature slowed the rate of metabolism, leading to much less brain damage.

The wear of an anxious, sleepless night showed on the faces of the house staff. Added to the strain of an evening and night of constant monitoring of their small charge, was the dawning realization that their efforts were futile. The many discussions had carried an inescapable message. All of us knew that the mild temperatures of Canon did not augur well for this child who had been discovered face down in the water by one of her parents. I watched her slow death-like respirations, very much like those of my former surgical patients. However, unlike patients under anesthesia, she made no signs of recovery. The endotracheal tube rose rhythmically. Her eyes were taped shut.

"How is she this morning?" Dan, a tall thin priest with curly, uncontrolled blond hair and a long, pointed, but surprisingly soft nose. He was the first year resident and ran work rounds.

"About the same as last night." Francisco, who always had something funny to say, said somberly.

"She's not waking up, huh?"

"No." Francisco, who liked to be called Frank, looked at the floor. We moved on slowly as a half-slumbering herd of beasts.

□ □ □ □

Two days later. Work rounds. The tiny body lay on a crisp white sheet as the pediatricians entered the Peds I.C.U. The medical students were allowed to touch, just touch, the little girl who but for a faint heart beat showed no signs of life. That we were allowed this close to the patient, that they did not fear that we might harm their small charge represented a change in the attitude of the priests of the Child God. It showed, as the somber expressions on their faces, that the little girl was already beyond the skill of the priests of the God of Life. It was strange that the student-priests, so eager to be allowed access to any pediatric patient, shunned prolonged contact with this patient. Our avoidance of the little girl was not meant to impress the house staff with our restraint and thereby extract more responsibility for us. No, it was something more akin to the prolonged and obligatory hand washing after an unsuccessful attempt to revive the victim of a cardiac arrest. We were avoiding any connection with the causation of the obviously terminal course of this patient. We were uncomfortable with death, particularly in a child. We saw for the first time the markedly proscribed limits of the power of priests.

The discussions of the house staff grew increasingly morbid.

"Any change?" Dan, the first year resident asked. His tone, which on previous days had rang with concern, was matter of fact.

"She's becoming a little more acidotic." Francisco answered.

"What are your plans with her?" Marty Boyer asked. He was the, seldom seen, pediatric Chief Resident who had just joined morning rounds.

Dan, the first year resident with curly blond hair answered him. "Just maintain her right now."

"Is she waking up?" There was a didactic point to the Chief resident's question. The Chief was acting as guide to the junior resident-priest.

"No." Dan, looked discomforted by the question.

"It's been how many days now?"

"Three."

"And she's not waking up at all?"

"No, not at all." Dan fidgeted. "We've talked with the family. We've explained to them what her condition is. They still say they want everything done." There was anguish and frustration in the resident's voice.

"You told them she would be a vegetable even if she survives."

"Yes."

"I see." The chief resident nodded knowingly, sympathetically. Marty was satisfied that the junior resident had asked the right questions even if his hands were tied. We moved on to the next patient.

Later that day a "Code Blue", the code word for a cardiac arrest, was called in the Pediatric ICU. The student-priests knew without being told who had coded, just as we knew that the priests-in-training welcomed their often adversary, Death. For in this case continued life would have been a cruel task master.

CHAPTER 32

Though we are well-heeled in the healing arts, we can effect no cures till we ourselves are open to solace and self-healing.
--Academy lectures

To those of you who may be new to this series, let me take a moment to tell you what it's all about. Several months ago, we decided that we needed a format with which we as physicians and nurses could look at the psycho-social aspects of medical care and critically assess the coping mechanisms of patients and their families. So, once a month we bring in an interesting outside speaker to discuss different aspects of the psycho-social part of patient care.

"Today we're going to talk about what I consider a failure in the treatment of one little girl, Letitia Jackson, and particularly the problem with her mother.

"We don't have a full-time pediatric gastroenterologist on staff here. Although I am not a gastroenterologist, I was called upon to supervise Letitia's care.

"Over the several months Letitia stayed here the staff of 8-West grew unusually close to her . . . "

“The whole hospital did." a young nurse with short-cropped hair interrupted the priest whose beard was speckled with gray. He continued.

"When one puts a lot of emotional and intellectual energy into a patient's care, one hopes for a good result at least. None was forthcoming in Letitia's case. The frustration and pain we all felt was not made better by the relationship with Letitia's mother. No one was able to form any kind of relationship with the child's mother. Not any physician, any nurse, not a single person. She distrusted us all." The priest's voice trailed off into a bitter silence.

"You know, she always felt that we were not doing all that we could for Letitia." The head nurse, a solidly built woman with dark brown, almost black hair spoke. "I guess since we could not find out what was wrong with her, it probably did seem that way to her."

"That's true." The priest was back again. "She had a progressively down-hill course and did not get better no matter what we did. Even to the end we did not know what was making her ill."

"Didn't the mother bring in some kind of faith healer or something to exorcise the evil spirits that were enchanting her daughter."

"By the time Letitia left, the house staff was ready to call in an exorcist to figure out what was wrong with her."

"Yeah, didn't the mother start putting things in Cora's food that the healer gave her?"

"We thought that that might be the case, but we were never able to prove it." The priest with gray in his beard interjected.

The confessions of the nurses and priests continued.

"You know she did talk to one person, though."

"Who?"

"She talked to Josie. Is Josie here?"

"No, she's off today." The mood became a little less restrained

"Where was the father during all of this?"

"Gone."

"Gone?"

"He was a serviceman who married Letitia's mother somewhere overseas, then brought her over here."

"She wasn't American?" The guest speaker, a short pleasant, plump psychologist in her mid-forties spoke for the first time.

"No, she was Filipino, wasn't she?" The head nurse looked around the room as she spoke. No one knew for certain.

"That puts a different light on things." The psychologist spoke again. "But what about the father?"

"The father left three months after bringing the family over here. Letitia was only a few months old when he left them."

"The mother hated Americans."

"After what the father did to her, small wonder." The psychologist interjected.

"I never knew that." The graying priest spoke as if awakened from a trance. The struggle within himself showed clearly upon his face.

"Knew what?"

"That she hated all Americans."

"Yes, that was quite clear with her talks from Josie. She hated all Americans with a vengeance." The head nurse spoke.

The lines of tension eased in the face of the graying priest. His personal solution to the long vexing enigma of Letitia's mother was given to him. With the answer, he found a small piece of peace. The guest psychologist wisely seeing that the time was one of venting long pent up feelings, not analysis, said little as the river of emotion raged then dissipated into a sea of silence.

Later, an attending priest, hair the color of smoke-laden gold, spoke of a child he had taken care of several years before as a house officer. He had called the parents to get the child who was then well. The mother had said that she would have to wait until the father got home from work. An accident occurred whereby the child slipped from a high chair and choked to death. The priest was faced with the task of telling the parents that their daughter, who was perfectly well two hours before, was dead.

Another quiet space passed after the telling of the priest's tale. Then, as the hour was up, the social workers, nurses, priests, and aids of 8-West, comrades-in-arms in the fight against human suffering, filed out of the room, somber, but uplifted as they had won a small victory for themselves.

THE THIRD YEAR

CHAPTER 33

. . . when you smile, I feel warm inside.
—an unsung poet.

The extraordinary luck I have had finding companionship, during the few times I have actively sought it impresses me with the pervasiveness of loneliness. It is a malady as old and as universal as the tread of human tears on human faces. It is as inseparable from humanity as loving, caring, hunger, or dying. It is a universal truth that makes we humans paradoxically social creatures.

Enter Aisha. When I think of her I believe that some power beyond human reason does exist and sent her to me to give me a respite, if ever so brief, from loneliness, to give me the strength to accomplish just a bit more with my life. She boarded the bus, clad in a worn, tweed sport coat and her fingers thrust deep into the pockets of a pair of faded, comfortable-looking jeans. Her hair was worn in a short Afro.

"Does this bus go to State?" She asked, referring to the State College.

"Yes." the driver, a short man with prematurely grave features answered.

She handed him a piece of paper, a transfer. For a moment she stood, near the door, just beyond the well-manicured vehicle operator. She moved uncertainly. I regarded her calmly. She saw me, looked past me, then continued. She stopped suddenly, swung into the seat in front of mine.

"Do you know what time it is?" She spoke to me. My wrist was bare. "I'm sorry," I said, "I don't have a watch."

"Dog, I sure hope I get there before eight . . . Excuse me, " she called to another passenger, "Do you know what time it is.?"

A short dark-skinned man looked beneath the sleeve of his coat. "Yeah, it's seven-o-three."

"Thanks."

"You going to State?" I asked.

"Yeah."

"This bus will get you there about three minutes before eight." She looked relieved. "Are you going to see Dick Gregory by any chance.?"

"Yeah." she answered. "That where you going?"

"Oh, yes." I answered.

"Oh, good. Do you know where he's going to be at?"

"Montezuma Theater as I remember, but don't ask me where that is." I introduced myself.

Her name, she told me, was Aisha. "Aisha." I repeated tentatively.

"Yes," she went on, "she was the wife of Mohammed."

"She was the mother of Fatima who married Ali wasn't she?" I asked excitedly. "Ali was the first leader of the Shiite sect of Islam."

The blank expression on her face told me that she knew nothing of the things I spoke. We passed a time of pleasant small talk as the bus ground slowly across the city of canyons.

A few years previously at my undergraduate college, I had heard Dick Gregory speak. Though he was a national celebrity, I had wavered over whether or not to see him. Finally, I had decided in favor of going, more out of boredom than anything else. I had been thoroughly impressed that though he had been billed as simply a comedian, that he was in truth a consummate political analyst and a man whose humanity and love ran as deep as the womb of the inky blue sea. He was funny, but beyond the humor was an angry, impassioned man who saw America as it was, yet maintained an unfailing belief that it could change and attain the greatness of its ideals.

I followed as a child behind the domineering and lovable Aisha as she walked toward a few empty seats about half way toward the front of the auditorium. Though, I usually resented domineering individuals, I must confess that I was both amused and charmed by Aisha. There was a basic goodness about her despite her rough and unpolished manner. I knew without her telling me that she was street-wise, that her life had been a hard one. Yet I knew also that she was sweet and gentle and kind.

Dick Gregory spoke of many things. He spoke of the temple of the body, that good minds began with good food and physical health. He spoke of the diseases of the heart which caused this great nation to slaughter blameless children in their homes. He spoke of a war waged openly by the United States, then another secret war which had caused him to take a vow which allowed him not one morsel of solid food for several years while the killing continued. He spoke of the environment, of our homes, our work places, our highways where every day another of us was struck down by the dreaded beast, cancer. He spoke of how by threatening a massive demonstration he had received a letter from the President of the United States in the space of a few hours. He spoke of constant surveillance by Government agencies, his virtual news blackout when he, nearing 40, had run the breadth of this nation. As he spoke, many, if not most, of his efforts were directed against the building of nuclear plants. A moment of quiet was called for as he told us of the death of a dear friend and traveling companion. We were sad with him. Finally, he gave us the opportunity to join with him in spirit. Every week from sunset Friday to sunset Saturday he fasted. He did this to remember those who slept with hunger rather than a pillow, those who were victims of disease, prejudice, injustice. I was deeply moved by the things that were said. I thought a long while in another world. When the lecture was over, Aisha and I, moved silently, soberly along walkways carpeted in red adobe. I needed a few moments of quiet reflection. I needed silence to think about the ideals of this man, leading a crusade against many of the evils of the world, ideals which I shared, but which had seemed to have lost their meaning of late. I seemed bent upon a course of selfishness, self-import, and it seemed at times self-abuse as well. Things had not always been that way. Perhaps for the space of ten minutes, I pondered over the things said by Gregory as Aisha and I walked without words. Having met only a few hours previously, ten minutes without speaking was not a long time--it was a life time. Aisha had also been quiet and contemplative. I felt a comfort with this woman that I had shared with few on this planet, especially any I had known for so a short time. I watched her face as we walked back to the bus stop, allowing her the space her eyes told me she needed. One A.M. found Aisha and I trekking across the city of canyons on a bus once more. The gentle rocking of her head against my chest where she had lain it was pleasurable. I was on-calling the next day. Somehow that caused me no concern as both the night and my company were pleasant. I waved good-by as the bus pulled noisily into gear. Waving back, she smiled warmly. I watched her face, brown and sleep-laden, disappear into the night as a quietness settled over the streets. Aisha. Was the magic in the name or the woman? My thoughts whispered gently again, Aisha.

CHAPTER 34

We play to remember in the times we forget how.

--a priest of the God of Children

Seven thirty-two A.M. I cringed as I tried to sneak by the clock. The group of a dozen people--interns, residents, nurses, medical students--stood in the room of the second patient. I joined them quietly, peering over the shoulder of one of the medical students. I looked with intent interest as the intern spoke. All my colleagues and a few of the priests, as well, watched the television screen. My late arrival and the lack of interest shown by the student-priests who were present as observers only had become all too familiar. We moved slowly, disjointedly to the next room. A small toddler with sandy-colored hair looked at us joyfully, jumping as we entered. The discussion of patients continued around the room. I stood toward the rear of the group, winking and waving at the little girl who enjoyed the attention. There was no television in the room. We moved on, quickly. We made our way around the back part of the U-shaped corridor, past the closed doorway to the ICU. We stopped in front of a room. A handsome boy, perhaps eight or nine, with smooth, round features watched us gloomily. The priests looked at the boy with saddened, knowing glances. The boy turned to look at the television.

"It's a shame what happened to that kid, huh?" Sally, the pathologist turned pediatrician offered.

"Yeah, it really is."

The boy mainly kept his eyes on the television, but stole an occasional glance at us.

Dan, the curly haired Nordic priest, spoke. "Maybe you should close the door. He can hear everything we're saying." Francisco pulled the large flat metal handle. The house staff spoke of a young boy, born and living in Mexico, who went to a surgeon in his home town because of an inguinal hernia. The hernia was operated on, however, a mishap occurred. The surgeon's blade partially transected the base of the boy's penis.

The urologists of the University Hospital had been called. They had been unable to ascertain the full measure of the damage, but had felt that while urination would probably be unaffected, sexual function would be impaired if not totally lost. This had been explained to the boy's family who had brought him to the American side of the border when they had noted the mishap.

"Does he know?" Sally asked.

"They have talked with him about it." Dan spoke.

"Even if he knows," Francisco, most often called Frank, interjected, "what would it mean to him at his age?" We all nodded in silent agreement. "All he knows is that his penis looks funny."

"That's really a shame." Sally spoke.

Dan pushed the door open. Our patient, who had been sitting on the bed before, was nearly struck by the door as we entered. He cut off the light in the bathroom which was immediately adjacent to the room's entrance. As he made his way back to his bed, I wondered how long had he been there and how much had he heard? The bed bobbed up and down gently as he sat. He regarded us with only a mildly anxious equanimity. His expression remained sad, somber.

"Good morning, Eugenio. You feel O.K. this morning?" Dan spoke to the young boy.

The boy nodded yes to no one in particular.

"Hablas Inglés?" (Do you speak English?) Frank called to the boy in Spanish.

"Yes, he speaks English." Dan answered.

Eugenío gave a single grave nod of his head, indicating that he did indeed speak English. This time he looked directly at Francisco.

Dan continued. "Any problems with urination, with making pee-pee?"

He shook his head no. As Dan continued with the interview, I found my eyes falling slowly toward the small out-pouching in the space between his legs. It was only with great effort that I was able not to stare at this area of his anatomy. With great perseverance, Dan was able to extract two monosyllabic replies after about five questions.

Despite the boy's calm exterior, fear resided deep within the brownness of his eyes. We left the room without examining our patient. I was grateful that the priests of the Child God showed consideration for the boy's feelings, but I was just as deeply disappointed that I was not able to witness the cruel caprice of the God of the Knife. As we continued, each of us paused a moment to thank our respective Gods that we had not been dealt so brutal a blow.

CHAPTER 35

Love is an ever-precious gift though it be
at times fleeting and clothed in pain.
--unknown poet

The afternoon sky was clear save for a single billowed cloud. As we made our way to my home, my thoughts were on cooking. I worried as I wanted the meal to be special. Most of the day, a Sunday, had been passed at a community art center. The myriad of objects on display, dancing, and drama had held our attention well into the afternoon and had led us to change our minds about a contemplated movie. Besides, Aisha confessed that she was starved. Our decision on the spur of the moment to go downtown before the dinner I was to prepare had cut short some last-minute shopping needed for the meal. I was feeling the slight pressure of time.

As I opened the door, the solid and reassuring quietness of my apartment, my shelter from the storms of life, greeted me as an old friend. I took Aisha's sweater. She immediately, irrevocably fell in love with my bean bag chair, insinuating herself in its folds before the television.

I smiled, quickly going about the business of preparing dinner--chicken sautéed with tomatoes, mushrooms, and garlic, fresh corn and rice. For dessert, I made a fresh fruit salad. This last item, I knew Aisha would like as she was very much a lover of natural foods. I busied myself in the kitchen. How long was the food going to take? she asked impatiently. I asked if she were one of those guests who pestered her host all night with such questions? She did not reply. I heard nothing from her until I was making the fruit punch. I felt her warmth at my side. "Hm-m-m. What do you call this?" She indicated the main course.

"I don't really have a name for it. How about chicken-a-la-George?"

She smiled as she tasted the entree. Pleasant surprise showed on her face. "Goo-o-od." She crooned. Her smile spread. Something clicked as she stood before me. I slid my arm around her waist, pulling her warm woman body next to mine. I kissed wonderfully soft brown lips. A secret joy rushed through my body that I wanted never to end.

"You keep on doing that and you ain't going to never eat." I teased.

She laughed. We kissed again. She took a second sample of the chicken. Slowly with a walk that exuded sensuality, she returned to the living room. I watched her as she settled comfortably back into the bean bag chair.

Good food, good company. What more could a man ask for? Dinner was superb. I was delighted with fruit of my efforts. We settled into the living room to eat as my kitchenette had no table. We ate contentedly, leisurely.

After dinner, we discussed the imposing, three by four-foot painting which dominated my living room. I was proud of the portrait which had taken me six weeks working on it daily. My first oil painting, it was something of both beauty and permanence. I always meant to point it out to my guests, but my visitors usually noticed it before I remembered to say anything.

"Where did you find that painting? I've been looking for something like that."

She felt good in my arms--warm soft, and full of a wonderful womanliness. I looked within her brown eyes. Talking about my painting was not what I wanted to do just then. "I did it."

"You did it?"

"Yes." I nodded.

"And the words?"

"Mine, also."

She looked at the painting, mouthing the words. It was a simple yet beautiful poem which told of the aspirations of a man, a dreamer. She read the final line aloud. "That's nice." She commented.

"Not as nice as you." I said as I brought my face close to hers. My smiling lips and hers mingled together in a sea of lush warmth. I knew after this kiss that we would make love. The intensity, the feeling with which she kissed me, her body language, all were to me unequivocal. I languished in the joy of her embrace. The affection which I so desperately needed had seemed so far and now within the arms of Aisha I had an overabundance of it. I wanted, needed her desperately. My hands held her waist tightly.

"That's ENOUGH!" She said sharply. Her words were a stinging slap. I had planned the dinner to be a meal, no more. When we had kissed in the kitchen, it had been something that just happened, something totally spontaneous.

What had come after had come with her permission and participation. I stared back at her dumbly. Was this simply a ploy? Something in her voice, her sudden change in manner told me that it was not that kind of a game and to press the issue would be to lose everything, including her friendship.

I began to feel a deep hurt as rejection, once again, reared its ugly head. I felt I had been tricked, my emotions played with. I felt anger.

I excused myself. Closing the bathroom door behind me, I began to try and put my tumbling thoughts in order. I could not. Deep hurt dominated my thinking. I must, at least, play the part of the good host. I avoided looking at Aisha as I returned to the living room. I could feel her eyes follow me as I moved toward the record player. An album fell onto the turn table.

“You know, you're going to have learn to deal with rejection. You can't get so upset because a girl tells you 'no:'"

"Really?!"I answered testily. "What makes you think I'm so upset?" I tried to put on my best poker face. It was an ineffectual effort. Anger had me firmly in its grasp. I picked up the dishes we had eaten in and busied myself in the kitchen.

"I'm sorry," her tone, still argumentative, was softer, much softer, "but I don't go to bed on the first date anymore."

There was something about the word "anymore" that cut through my anger like a knife. I turned toward her. For a brief moment, I could see beyond Aisha's street-tough veneer. The pain of too many relationships with cruel, self-serving men, the pain of a thousand lonely nights when she had cried herself to sleep were written clearly across her face. It was the only time in my brief relationship with Aisha that I could see the extent of her hurting and the depth of the scars it had left. Anger gave way to pity then to utter confusion.

Somehow, someway, I do not know how, we found one another's arms again that night. We spoke calmly. The urgency in my body dissipated. A time of fearful dread was followed by a calming quietness. After seeing Aisha to the bus stop, I lay in my room. The moon, pale and full, cast its white beams upon my spread. As I stared thoughtfully at the ceiling it came to me that the three of us would be sharing my bed once again--the moon, the emptiness, and me.

CHAPTER 36

Wisdom and courage are universal.
--the Heretic Priest

I **descended** the stairs, disappointed and somewhat forlorn. Aisha was not home. Ramses ascended the stairs, dressed crisply, stylishly in dark brown slacks and a shirt printed in subdued shades of lighter and darker brown. His long slender limbs, close cut Afro, and chiseled features would have made him at home in the fashion section of any magazine.

"What's happening?" I said with little feeling.

"HI!" Ramses spoke elated. "How you doing today?" Before I could answer, he continued. "You shouldn't scare people that way." He looked at me earnestly. What I had mistaken for gladness had been relief. Ramses had been scared witless.

"Really?" I answered, a smile crossing my lips.

"Shoot. I didn't know who you was, coming out of there like that. You should at least make some noise or something." I laughed aloud. Ramses smiled. Ramses lived in Aisha's building. We had spoken briefly a few times. "Where you say you go to school at?"

I called the name of the priest academy, then asked, "You're at State, aren't. you?"

"Yeah, but not for long."

"When do you leave?"

"In August."

"Where is it you said you were going?"

He called the name of a college I was not familiar with.

"Where's that?"

"It's about a hundred miles north of San Assisi." He continued with barely time for a breath. "They have a good program there in counseling?" I knew Ramses wanted to do counseling. "Oh, yes. Very good and very hard to get into, too. It's way out in the country, not near no big cities. You know, people ask me why I wanted to be out there so far from everything? But, you know, I'm going there to study. Out there, where there ain't no people always bothering you, saying 'come, let's do this, let's do that', I can really study."

"There's some really beautiful country up there." I added.

"Oh yeah. They have so much land, you won't believe. Somebody just gave them acres and acres. *Too much* land. When I went up there last month, I got lost. I asked the bus driver where to get off at, and he just told me he don't get paid for giving out information."

"Really?!"

"Yeah. I said 'How you going to drive a bus and not give out information?' I just walked for miles, then I got on another bus and that bus driver told me how to get to the man's office for my interview. You know something else?"

"No, what?"

"I didn't see another single Black person while I was there?"

"Humph"

"Yeah, but I don't let that bother me. I'm only going there to learn. No matter how they treat me." He paused for only a fraction of a second. "They ain't got too many Black folks where you at either, do they?"

I never stopped being amazed at how wide spread was the knowledge of the Academy's lack of Black and Brown students. "No, not many at all."

Ramses looked distantly before him. "Sometimes life is hard. You know, people sometimes make fun of me because I'm neurotic, have a few problems. People look at me, see me in these nice clothes, they wonder how come I don't have a car. But, you know, my parents was going to buy me a car, but it wasn't what I want. I want a Jaguar. You know, I don't want to settle for second best. If I can't have what I want, I don't want anything. So, I told them to just wait till they could give me what I want. So, they going to give me a Jag for graduation. "But I'm trying to keep it together until I finish school."

"I hear you there." I interjected.

"You know the only reason I'm living here is so I can pay my therapist. So, I figure I can live a little less extravagantly if going to him helps me deal with my problems. You know, before you counsel people, you got to have your own head together. You may think I'm crazy now, but I used to be a lot worse." (I smiled.) "I was strung out on everything there was. I used to sell it, too. If it wasn't for the girl I used to go with, I wouldn't be here right now. She saved my life. Twice I was dead. My heart had stopped beating and everything. Two times I overdosed and she found me unconscious, in a coma. Both times my heart stopped beating in the hospital and they started pumping on my chest and brought me back to life. After the second time, I said no more. No more drugs for me. All I do now is drink a little wine. Sometimes when things is hard, I just go up to my room by myself, lock the door, get me a glass of wine and play the same record over and over again by Chaka Khan--"Everybody's got an aura," and I keep myself together." In the moment's silence that ensued, I wondered how long had it been since I had kept myself together as I listened to a record make ribbons of a night that seemed as a shroud about to envelope me. How many years? It seemed like lifetimes ago, when I, like Ramses, had stood before myself in the cruelly honest mirror of my mind and found that I could bring me through the torment, albeit painfully, which always seemed worse at night.

We said our good-byes. As I descended quietly to the first floor, the sound of my steps on the carpeted staircase echoed noisily.

CHAPTER 37

I am gentle. I am hard. I am love.
--the Earth Poet

The night was pregnant with impending rain. The air, thick and heavy, stifled me as I sat in the sullen stillness of my living room. I dialed Aisha's number, quickly, almost automatically. The empty, unanswered ringing of the phone sounded an impotent challenge against a mounting restlessness. The record I placed on the turn table did nothing to ease the growing anxiety. Barely taking the time to throw on a denim jacket, I leaped on my bike and was down the stairs before the screen door closed. The beating of the ball bearings sounded fast and furious over oil-stained asphalt. I pedaled faster until the traffic lights, and the faces of passers-by blended into a soft blur. The surface of the streets, shining with condensed moisture, reflected street lamps which appeared as mottled gray moons in a bedraggled sky. I rode swiftly, to cover the several blocks between Aisha's home and mine. I rode faster to arrive before the falling rain. I rode faster yet, trying to outdistance the impenetrable gloom which was slowly overtaking me. My bicycle stopped abruptly in front of Aisha's house. She was not home, I knew. I crept stealthily over the stairs. I knocked at her apartment. No light could be seen under the door. No sound was heard within. I knocked a little louder. No one answered.

What to do now? Should I do the sensible thing and go or should I wait for heaven only knew how long? There was the slight groan of wood as I sat on the blind stairwell next to Aisha's door. Downstairs, the front door opened. Tired steps ascended the stairs. A man carrying a small grocery bag shuffled to the far end of the hall, unaware of my presence.

The rapid beating of my heart was stilled by bitter disappointment.

Several more people came in. After a time, I no longer looked. Two hours passed. A voice was heard indistinctly. Footsteps rose slowly. It occurred to me that Aisha was not coming home, that she was spending the night at a friend's. The hour was getting late. I knew I must leave soon. Two figures, a man and a woman, turned at the head of the stairs, coming toward me. The woman's voice became clear--it was Aisha's. Feelings of joy, embarrassment, relief, and discomfort battled within me. I looked from Aisha to her companion to Aisha again.

"Hi!" Aisha's tone was pleasant. She did not seem put out by my presence.

"Hi." I said, feeling awkward. I rose, throwing my overnight case behind me. "I just dropped by to say hello." My nervousness belied the forced casualness of my tone.

"Been here long?" She asked, still pleasantly. I did not answer the question. Impatience began to grow on the face of her companion.

"I don't want to impose. I'll see you another time," I told her.

"No, why don't you come in?" She sounded genuine. The door was open.

The three of us went inside. She introduced her companion. I made small talk for the space of two minutes while I tried to size up the situation. I came to no decision. I knew only that I did not know what was going on. Her companion looked over Aisha's apartment. told her that he liked it. I stood where I had entered, by the door, bag slung over my shoulder. "I know you have company. I really do have to go." I spoke to Aisha.

"No, stay." She protested. "He's leaving in a minute." She indicated her companion. I stayed where I was. He said his good-byes and left.

"So," she said looking me in the eye, "how was your day?"

"It was O.K." I answered. "Look, I'm sorry if my coming by unannounced got in the way of things."

"Oh, him?" She turned toward the kitchen. "I wanted him to see the apartment. He's thinking about moving." She went on to explain that she had met him only a few hours ago at a lecture at one of the local colleges and had begun talking as he gave her a ride home. She had shown him the apartment as she wanted to get a few "good" people to move into the building. She wanted to know what I was carrying in the bag. "We-ell, I needed someone to talk to." I said hesitating half a second. " a-and I was taking you up on your offer to spend the night."

The anger which I had convinced myself was not there flashed clearly across her face. "George," her voice was hard, cutting, "you're trying to crowd me."

I said nothing. I was incapable of saying anything. I was hurt very deeply. The full force of her fury rose. "I don't want to see you all the time. I don't want you calling me every day. I don't want you hanging around here."

Silence lay heavily between us.

"Look," her voice softened, "you can sleep on the extra bed if you want to."

"That's O.K." It was all I could do to muster a little anger. I did not feel it. All I felt was hurt. "I'll be going." It was beginning to rain.

"Bye!" she said, the hardness returning to her voice.

"Bye." I said softly, looking intently at the floor. I closed the door. Racing down the stairs, I did not look up again until I was well into the night. The rain fell onto my face blending its wetness with my own.

I had lost a foot race with gloom. I was overcome by hurt, loneliness, hopelessness, and despair. Sometime during the night, before the coming of dawn, I was enfolded, forgivingly, in the restful arms of sleep.

CHAPTER 38

Grant us courage.

--prayer of the priests of the God of Life

The sparrows conducted their morning business, noisily. I arose and showered. I arrived nearly on time as usual, before the house staff as usual, before work rounds as usual. I had decided to go to work, continue my daily routine.

Rounds moved into a room on the north side of the building. Eight stories above the ground, we had a panoramic view of Canon. The house staff began to discuss a case. Two of the medical students watched a morning talk show. I looked through the window at the city below. Somewhere in my mind George Benson crooned "Everything Must Change" in an almost ghost-like voice. I thought of the song's words. The piano solo, the baddest piano in the whole world, began playing. The notes, the keys, the fingers rippled through my soul, touched my pain. I wanted to fly. Like a big bird, I wanted to spread my wings out and feel the rushing wind against my face. The piano was there. I could hear every note like the piano was there in the room with me. I held on to the piano. The chords eased the hurt, soothed pain which was as a tense infected boil on my brain. Benson came back landing, gliding just behind the piano. But he was right, everything must change including the hurt I felt now that I knew that what was between Aisha and I was over. The discussion on rounds now centered around the care of a little girl, a toddler who smiled as we gathered around her crib. I listened attentively. How dare she treat me that way? I had spent a restless night wrestling with thoughts of Aisha. A voice within me, calm and undeniable spoke. She had only done what I had allowed her to do.

I dialed her number as the first gray rays of dawn entered my window. The ringing ended much too soon as she said hello. An unreasoned shouting began. She told me she did not care. I called her unfeeling. Expletives fell as rain drops on the night I had left her house. Finally, when all had been said, there was the mad race to hang up. She won. My vehemence still not expended, I picked up the phone and cursed the empty dial tone.

□ □ □ □

The chairman of the department spoke slowly, wisely—dully. Across from me, Sally's eyes stared vacantly at the empty chair before her. The piano was back in my mind.

A second case was presented. Jennifer's high-pitched, squeaky voice rose. For the first time that day, I could look at Aisha's words, my words, our relationship without the over-powering urge to flee. I wondered again, how could I have allowed myself to be so treated? The discordant, yet melodic clanging of the keyboard broke through, demanding an answer from a place where there was none. How could I have stopped it any sooner than I did? was a question more fair to me. As the chairman discussed the second case, he did not notice a lone student-priest sitting in the corner, clinging desperately to a piano.

CHAPTER 39

Courage when we have lost, shows an honor which is greater than any defeat.
--the Heretic Priest

Afternoon. University Hospital. Pediatrics.

"I have an interesting case you might like to see."

"Oh, really?" I answered.

"Yes." David continued, "the little kid in the crib in the corner." David was a fourth-year medical student, doing a sub-internship in pediatrics. He was both knowledgeable and likable. "Probably the mother had rubella during pregnancy. He was born deaf and is probably blind, in both eyes."

"Wow." I said.

"Yeah. A real tragic case."

"Indeed, it is." I answered. I made a mental note to return to the crib to examine the baby. It was near the end of the day. David left after writing a few orders. A beautiful afternoon with a clear azure sky and whispers of red clouds shone through the eighth-floor windows. It would have been a wonderful afternoon in which to do something fun with someone dear. I had neither the someone or the something. I would enjoy the ride home. Perhaps, later I would ride to the park and watch the joggers. I made my final rounds, checking on all my patients, looking to see if anything interesting was taking place on the floor. I entered the last room of the U-shaped corridor.

None of my patients were there. No procedures were taking place. The baby David had spoken of was in one of the cribs in the room. Another day, I thought.

The magic of the early autumn day grew strong enough to touch even my depressed spirits. It would be a nice day for soaking up some sun.

Parents milled around with their children. As I turned to leave, a face caught my eye, carrying me back to my days as an undergraduate. Rose. Yes, it was Rose.

Rose. The name walked through my mind in colors crimson and gold, winter breeze on an autumn afternoon. There were many good memories with that name, memories associated with a dozen girls named Rose who came into my life. I remember a girl in junior high school with short pressed hair who teased me as often as she called my name. I remember, in high school, another girl whose personality bubbled into my life. I remembered a zany girl in my homeroom. I remember a girl in college I would see seldom, one of two Roses in my network of friends. But the Rose before me was one for whom both I and Theodore had a special fondness, a girl who always greeted me with a smile, whose warm southern accent always delighted. I remembered her from my freshman Biology class. She had a grin that was at once unabashedly girlish and knowingly sophisticated. I remember my fondness for this Rose matched by that of Theodore. I remember seeing her across campus with Theodore.

He was physically similar to me, but younger looking, heavier-built, and his face yet imbued with the innocence I imagined long lost in mine. They had made a beautiful couple. She was brown-skinned, shapely, strangely graceful. He was tall with features handsomely shaped from the dark, hand-rubbed wood of west African sculptures.

I remember having felt jealous that he had spoken before I of the fondness we shared for the gentle smile, the quiet conversation with her. Perhaps his longing to be with her had been deeper than my own for it had prompted him to speak while I had found excuses for silence. While nothing had quieted my heart, my tongue was stilled by my loyalty to Theodore. I had believed in loyalty above all things then. Loyalty alone would have been enough to quiet my tongue.

While Theodore had given recklessly of his heart, Rose was more cautious, giving her affection in such a way as to make its recipient unsure of its meaning. It had not been long before I first saw Rose with Frank, the boyfriend of Vida. Many a jealous scene ensued. Soon Frank and Rose were a regular couple. However, as this relationship developed there was no clean break with Theodore.

Instead, she gave him just enough to keep him coming back. Pain rose slowly in Theodore's face as he came to realize the truth. I had hurt for both Theodore and myself as his fate could easily have been my own.

All these memories and more flowed through my mind as I saw Rose's face bathed in the glow of the afternoon sun at the University Hospital. A smile crossed my lips. I was very glad to see her. "Hey, what's happening?" I called out across the room. She smiled that same girlish, yet sophisticated smile of hers as I approached. "Hi!" she answered in a warm voice. Notwithstanding fine lines of worry, the six years since our last meeting had made only the barest imprint upon her face. She held a small child in her arms, feeding it from a bottle.

I approached Rose. We laughed and talked easily about times and friends past.

"Is that yours?" I asked. I referred to the baby in her arms.

"Yes."

"What is it?"

"A little boy."

"What's his name?" I asked as I placed my finger in his hand. He played with it contentedly. Rose uttered the child's name, a melodic grouping of Swahili words. The last name was English. "So that's your name now?" I repeated the baby's surname.

"No, that's his father's name. We're not married. You probably know him. He goes to the University." She told me his first name. The affection she had for the baby's father showed clearly.

"No, I don't think I know him." The baby manipulated my hand at will. "Tell me, what is he doing here?" I indicated the child in her arms.

"He can't see. They think he may have trouble with his hearing, too."

I looked closely at the infant. His skin was dark brown as were his eyes. His hair was jet black with opulent loose curls. It had seemed that the baby looked from mouth to mouth as Rose and I had spoken. However, as I looked again, more closely, I was not sure. Indeed, the more I looked, the less certain I became.

"We're really worried about him?" Concern was etched into her face.

"I can imagine. Perhaps these things will get better." I offered lamely.

"I sure hope so." I gazed at baby for a time. "Rose, what does his name mean?"

"His first name means 'conqueror.' His middle name means 'one who leads.'" The pride on her face touched me. The plight of both the parents and child made me realize that I had much in this life for which to be grateful.

Rose and I spoke again of old friends and what had become of them. When I left her that afternoon, the Sun had added crimson and gold to the brown flesh tones of her face, just as it had years before, but there was also a sadness there, deeper than time and more abiding.

CHAPTER 40

Life holds no greater mystery than its creation from the coupling of man and woman.

--Priests of the God of Fertility

The morning was overcast enough only to take the edge off the coldness as I climbed atop my red three speed bicycle. The group of students to which I was assigned was scheduled to do its Obstetrics-Gynecology rotation at Junipero Serra Hospital, a rambling, unplanned maze of buildings and walkways. The compound, from a time when aesthetics waged a losing battle with the technocracy of function, fell pitifully short of both goals. Having neither beauty nor utility to justify its existence, it slid un-consoled and irretrievably into depression and decay. The enfeebled miscellany of rusted iron, plaster, and wood withstood its irrevocable and immediate demise each day only by the determined and unflinching will of those who joined in the battle against human disease and suffering.

The cool magentas of dawn blended imperceptibly with the pink wall which formed the outer perimeter of Serra. Only the white-uniformed guard who nodded perfunctorily as I passed evinced that the hospital was a major naval installation. It was five minutes to six.

Morning rounds began promptly at six. The chief resident of Gynecology had warned us sternly that lateness was not tolerated.

In the two days I had traveled this early morning route I had arrived at the appointed hour, only to wait twenty to thirty minutes until the first intern or resident showed. The first morning I had paced the halls frantically, certain that I had misunderstood the directions given me and that the rest of the GYN house staff was rounding in another part of the hospital. Only the repeated reassurances of an amused and seasoned nurse had kept me from searching the grounds. The second day I was again the first to arrive, however, by the time the house staff showed up I was already checking patients.

I secured my bike quickly. At seven minutes after six, arrived on a ward that was quiet except for the soft tread of the night nurses making their final check before the change of shift. No doctors were present. I picked up the charts of the two patients whom I had seen and admitted the day before with Summerfield, the resident to whom I was assigned. I entered the room of the first patient. She was a twenty-eight year old female who had presented because of pain caused by an abscess of her left fallopian tube and ovary.

I touched the woman's foot gently to awaken her. "Good morning."

"Doc, its early." She stretched as she spoke.

"I know." I said. "How do you feel this morning?"

"O.K., I guess."

"Any pain?"

"A little. I had to ask the nurse for a shot." She yawned. "Nothing like it was yesterday."

"Let's take a look at your tummy." She tossed the sheet down to her upper thigh, then pulled the hospital gown up, exposing one breast, her entire abdomen, and most of her pubic area. I was very much discomfited by the unnecessarily wide exposure of flesh in this smiling, stretching young woman. My first reflex was to call a nurse to stand by. But, I reasoned, if I did that for every abdominal exam, I would not only become an unbearable burden to the nursing staff, I would also never get any work done. Besides I was certain that my reaction was engendered more by my unwanted celibacy than by any behavior by my patient. Before I began my exam, I replaced the sheet so that it covered the triangle of hair below her navel. The tenderness of the previous day indeed seemed much diminished as I pushed gently on her belly. I covered the remaining exposed skin. "We'll see you a little later."

The intern whizzed straight from the door to the chart rack. He flashed a smile at me. "Good morning."

"Good morning," I answered. He disappeared into a room. I continued on my own patient rounds. I saw the second patient I had admitted with Summerfield. She had prolonged and irregular bleeding and was scheduled for a diagnostic D & C. The student grapevine, that all permeable and amazingly accurate information system, had informed me that I should know everything about any patient I saw in the morning including past illnesses, surgeries and all medications they were on. Students not knowing this information were to be dragged through the mud. Accordingly, I had committed to memory all the pertinent data of my two patients.

Summerfield had told me that I was responsible only for new patients which we admitted together. Thus, I could follow a case from beginning to end. Six-twenty A.M. I had seen both my patients. A second doctor, dressed in the standard white navy uniform arrived. I sat poring over the charts of the two patients double checking every piece of lab data, every note which might yield an answer to any question. I scribbled a few new entries on my index cards. It was six-thirty. All the Navy docs, except Summerfield and the chief resident were present. Summerfield had several patients besides the two I followed. He was late and time was drawing short. I knew basically what was going on in the remainder of his patients, but not in the minute detail I knew I would need for morning report. I picked up another of Summerfield's charts. Given the half hour until rounds, I could check the patient and familiarize myself with the chart even enough for morning report. At least, Summerfield would have one less patient to see. I saw the patient. Six: thirty-seven. I sat memorizing the minutia on which I might be tested as Summerfield appeared. I told him that I had already checked my two patients as well as another of his. He thanked me. He grabbed the six remaining charts.

"Hey, what are you doing now?" he asked as I leafed through the chart. I told him. "You don't have to worry about that." I told him what the student grapevine had said about morning report.

"No-o-o," he crooned, "you don't have to worry about that kind of stuff at all."

"Well, if you say so." He divided the charts in his arm, handing half to me.

"Here, do me a favor. Help me out with these charts."

"Sure." I took the extended clip boards. I was glad to help him. He was likable. Seven o'clock came swiftly.

Seven: twelve. Marvin Shorely, the chief resident walked on to the ward at his usual hour. He wore navy whites and a green khaki jacket. He laid his brief case upon a long table. Almost all the house staff were assembled in the room, talking, writing notes, checking lab data.

"Come on let's start morning report," he called out. The noise remained at the same level. Norman Rollins, a short perky intern with short, dark brown hair and round, black-rimmed glasses, looked askance at the chief resident. Most of the house staff either ignored or had not heard him. A pen in the corner, Summerfield's, moved faster.

"Where's Campbell?" the chief resident was testy.

"He was waiting here before, but I think he went to get some coffee." Norman spoke with thinly disguised mockery.

The chief resident said nothing. A small, thin resident with what looked like the aftermath of near-terminal acne appeared. The chief resident pulled a stack of index cards from his shirt.

"Alright, let's begin." He called the name of a patient- A resident called out the findings on exam and new lab data. Shorely scribbled as the house officers below him spoke. He called a patient of Summerfield's. The resident spoke without looking up from the chart he was writing. A few more names were called. The name of another of Summerfield's patients was called. The patient was one I had not followed, but had checked that morning for Summerfield. The resident answered without looking up. "The student saw the patient." I was surprised. I had reported my findings to Summerfield.

The chief resident looked at me. His eyes narrowed. I began, uneasily, to give report on the patient as I had seen the house officers do. As a student, I knew I would have to give more detail. I could not say simply, "no change," as did the residents and interns. "Mrs. Jacobs was afebrile. The rest of her vital were normal."

"Wait a minute," interrupted the chief resident. I swallowed audibly. "We want to know something more about this patient." The corners of his mouth, habitually turned down in a thin tight-lipped half frown, turned upward in sadistic joy. "Why is this patient in the hospital?" I repeated by rote memory the name of the procedure she had undergone. He leaned forward, firing the second question before I had finished my answer to the first. "How many days post-op is she?" I did not remember the exact number. I searched through my cards. I could not find hers. I knew the patient had been in the hospital about two weeks. I told this to the chief resident. "Give me that chart." I handed the metal clip board to him. He flipped through the history and physical. "She's twelve days post-op. You should know the exact number of days." I looked at Summerfield. He looked pointedly at the wall, saying nothing. My mind went through names for Summerfield beginning with spineless and ending with a string of expletives. "What was her chief complaint on admission?"

What little poise and confidence I had had evaporated. "Lower abdominal pain." I looked at Summerfield again. He refused to look at me.

"How long she have it for?" Shorely fired. I did not know. He read the answer from the chart. "When was her last period?" I did not know. He fired a salvo of questions in such rapid succession that I had no time to answer, right or wrong.

"What medications is she on?" I told him. "When was the last dose?" I did not know. "How come you don't know?" I looked at Summerfield as I thought of still another expletive that fit him.

I spoke to the chief resident. "I am not following the patient."

"What do you mean you're not following the patient?" He looked at me through narrowed blue eyes. "You should know every patient on this ward." I was shaken. All present knew that his statement was nonsense. As chief resident he could not be expected to know the twenty-five to thirty-five patients on the ward at any given time in the detail he asked of me. To expect more from a third-year clinical clerk was ludicrous. He stared at me for a long second as if emphasis would make his statement more credible. The furrows of his brow extended into a scalp which lay exposed beneath a short crew cut.

He called another name. Morning report continued with no break in the cadence, but with a palpable under-current of tension. He called a few more names. Residents answered quickly. He called another name. There was a strained silence as Fred Hauser, the second student on Gynecology, shuffled through his cards nervously. The almost olive tones of his skin, accentuated by a sun which had thrown off the shackles of the dawn's grayness, belied his Germanic name. "Oh, yeah." he called out as he came to the card for the patient whose name had been called. "No temp, post-op day number . . . one. Abdomen is soft. Bowel sounds are present." Fred looked up. A tense half-second followed in which no one breathed. "Fine." The chief resident smiled at the student through wire-rimmed glasses. He called the next name. The iniquity of the chief resident's actions struck me as a physical blow for only the second time that morning.

□ □ □ □

The large clock in Serra park struck seven as I pedaled homeward. I was tired, hungry, dejected as the cold wind of my passing blew across my face. I stopped my bike on the narrow concrete bridge which spanned the steep gorge.

Many feet below me a highway curved over the valley floor. Lines of red and white marked the passage of cars which disappeared in a tangle of trees and asphalt. The house staff and my colleagues had gone home some three hours before. I fingered the cards in my pocket. I had spent the hours after work copying the information from twenty odd patients onto the three by five pieces of cardboard. I did not like being "pimped." (That was the name students gave to the perversion of the Socratic method as it had been used by the chief resident.) I had begun to memorize information from the often illegible charts. After spending the better part of an hour on the first two charts, I was impressed that my first estimation was correct. That I could not memorize all the information on all the patients and continue with my primary objective, learning, was ludicrous.

THE THIRD YEAR

A tired figure pushed on across the expanse of steel and concrete, unmindful of any movement in the pale and moonless night.

CHAPTER 41

There's a hole in me where you used to be.
--an unsung poet

If you two need someone to listen to you, I'll be glad to donate some time." Garret Frank spoke of Grace and I. I listened to him with an intensity which did not match my outer. casualness. He spoke preparatory to our delving into the planned business of the meeting, my thesis project. A phone call by my wife had prompted his offer. I listened, at first feeling piqued that Grace had discussed our marital problems with one of my professors, someone whom to her was a virtual stranger. I heard all that was said in the statement that cut so to the core of my life. With one sentence he said many things--that my marriage was failing, that he knew my marriage was failing, and that Ann had confided a great deal more information to him. In the subtlety of subtleties that always marked Dr. Frank's comments, I detected another message--that if I wanted, I could defer a decision on his offer. I could also flatly reject his offer. I chose to delay my answer.

I hummed a yes that said only that I was listening, had heard. I paused for less than the space of a second before plunging into the research which formed the core of my work. Frank took this in without so much as a knowing glance.

Two weeks later. I sat in Frank's office at the main campus. "You know, she's always been very dependent on me."

Dr. Frank listened attentively. He asked a question. "Are you sure *she* is the one dependent upon *you*?"

His question, no, his statement, demanded a reply. "Yes!" I blurted, gripping the arms of the chair.

Frank was totally unruffled, "You know, your wife doesn't strike me as being that dependent." He repeated, driving home the point.

I argued against his statement with emotion and vehemence. He was wrong. He was clearly wrong. He was unequivocally wrong.

Wasn't he?

CHAPTER 42

Procreation is the path to the eternal.
--a priest of the God of Life

The salmon-colored walls were tinted gold by the rising sun. I secured my bicycle quickly. I felt good after a restful night, ready for my first night of obstetrics call. I wore the shoulder strap of my black vinyl bag across my chest like the bandolero of a tall and ready warrior. Routine set in quickly as I saw my patients. I moved slowly, taking the full time allotted to me so that I would not be asked to see any patients I did not know. Fred Hauser, my colleague on gynecology, arrived in the middle of my rounds. He carried a pack with him. It looked very much like that in which he carried his over-night gear. As I completed my rounds, I saw Rich Picard and Patrick Stein,
making their way leisurely toward the delivery room. Obstetrics was not required to start as early as gynecology.

"Hi!" I hailed my classmates.

"Hi!" My colleagues returned my smile.

"How was call last night?" Dave asked me.

Call? Last night? "I was not on-call last night. I'm on call tonight."

As Pat shook his head, he gave me the same half-mocking, half-pitying look that he had given me when he found that I was to follow Rich on Urology. I had an empty sinking feeling in the pit of my stomach. "Fred's on call tonight."

I looked into the faces of both my colleagues. "No," I said.

They both nodded yes.

When they had gone, I looked for a schedule in the GYN conference room. The student-priests' schedule was not there. The only other place to look for a schedule was in a distant part of an adjacent building. The chief resident was due at any moment. I did not dare be absent when he arrived.

Uneasily, I sat through morning report. The priests broke for breakfast. I did not join them. Instead, I made my way furtively through a myriad of corridors and passageways. After several wrong turns, I stood at the entrance to a large conference room. Impatiently, I scanned the bulletin board until my eyes fell upon the familiar printing of the medical students' schedule.

I swallowed audibly. They were right. I had missed my on-call night. I looked up and down the corridor fully expecting to see accusing fingers pointing menacingly at me. Slowly, burdened with guilt at having shirked my responsibility and filled with trepidation for the consequences of my act, I made my way back to the GYN ward.

What to do now? I could not simply pretend it did not happen. Though the priests had said nothing, I was sure that my absence had not gone unnoticed. I decided that the best thing I could do was to tell Summerfield, the resident to whom I was directly responsible. Nervously, I awaited Steve's return, hoping that I would see no other priest.

"You were supposed to be on-call last night. No one saw you." A voice boomed from nowhere. I was taken back not by the anger in his voice, but by the easy familiarity with which he addressed me. I had never spoken to the priest, nor could I remember having seen him before. I looked into cold blue eyes burning through gold wire rimmed glasses.

"I . . . I" I stammered.

"Did you switch with someone or something?" The cold anger in his voice made it clear that he knew I had not switched with anyone. I wondered did the priest hope to catch me in a lie.

"I . . . I got my days mixed up." I answered lamely.

The priest's stare did not change.

"I thought I was on call tonight." I thought to offer my overnight bag, my black vinyl case, as evidence of my good intentions, but decided against it. There was a very long uncomfortable pause.

"I hope this won't happen again." The sandy haired priest spoke sternly.

"No . . . no, it won't." The priest's blue eyes burned into me once again. I looked at the floor. The priest marched past me, stiffly. It was several minutes after he had gone before I could raise my eyes.

□ □ □ □

A few minutes later, Summerfield arrived. I told him of my error, of my encounter with the sandy haired priest.

"A-a-aw, don't worry about it." Summerfield seemed unperturbed. I felt somewhat reassured as I followed my cheerful instructor in the rites of the God of Fertility. As I followed Summerfield to clinic, my mind wandered to a few days before when the I had been told the same words by the same priest. I began to worry—a lot!

CHAPTER 43

Bigotry is seldom practiced either consciously or with malevolence. One has but to listen to the lofty language of its practitioners, observe their intricate intellectualizations to realize that they believe their cause is just.

--the Heretic Priest on prejudice

G**uiltily, I struggled** to finish my half-eaten steak. Norman Rollins, an intern who was teased relentlessly because he bore the name of a famous United States Senator, pulled the chair opposite Summerfield. Norman's thick rimmed glasses made his eyes appear unnaturally, grotesquely large. The act of sitting down, like almost everything else the intern did, seemed to overwhelm him. His country boy mannerisms and deep southern accent made him stand out among his fellow priests though several of them were also from the South. He smiled politely, almost apologetically, as he sat down.

The short-statured priest rose quickly. "I forgot the bread." He muttered as trotted back to the serving area. He returned after a moment. "A meal is not a meal without bread." He spoke to Summerfield as he jabbed a folded column piece of white bread into a pool of oil-laden gravy. Summerfield smiled mockingly.

"Y'all got some surgery to do this afternoon?" Rollins asked.

Summerfield chewed on a piece of bread as he tore it into long strips. "A couple D & C's." He answered disinterestedly.

"I haven't had much time in the O.R. I'd be glad even for a few D. & C. 's"

"Don't worry, you'll get them. More than you want."

"I imagine you're right."

As he pushed another strand of bread into his mouth, the resident-priest studied the intern a bit more kindly. Norman looked into his plate thoughtfully as he stirred the oily gravy.

"What do you have this afternoon?" Steve asked the intern.

"O.B. clinic."

"What do you have after the D. & C.'s?"

"GYN clinic."

"I heard you had a real interesting case the other day," the intern remarked.

Summerfield who had been thawing slowly from an initial cold disdain began to warm rapidly. "Yeah, that was a good case."

"How did she present?"

The resident priest leaned toward the intern. He began in the classic fashion of the priests of the God of Fertility. "She was a thirty-one year old Flip. She was gravida five, para three, Ab two, I think . . . " Here the priest paused involuntarily. His eyes slowly came around to mine.

Flip? What the heck is a flip? Though I had never heard the term, I realized that the priest was giving a derogatory name for Filipinos. The guilt-ridden look on the resident-priest's face told me that I had guessed correctly.

I tried never to show priests I worked with my feelings toward instances of evinced racism as I felt this gave them an unwanted edge on how to apply pressure when they wanted to do so. Nonetheless, I am sure that anger and disgust were written as clearly on my face as guilt on that of the resident-priest.

Summerfield turned slowly back to the southern priest who somehow had missed the entire transaction. He looked intently at the boyish face of the intern while he continued. I left quietly, saying nothing to either.

CHAPTER 44

The control of fertility is an issue central to our existence. It is a conduit of power, a major anchor point on which all important decisions must directly or indirectly impact.
--the Heretic Priest

She was twenty-three, an OR technician at Serra, attractive, Black, a patient on the GYN ward, and advertising single. I was twenty-five, a student on GYN, hurting, and lonely. She gave me subtle come-on's, signals that she would enjoy more than the patient physician relationship that I strictly adhered to. I enjoyed talking to her, enjoyed the commonness of shared experiences of fellow travelers in an oft times hostile world, rejoiced in our Africaness, and our dedication to serving the afflicted. Also, I was a student-priest in an order whose origin could be traced to the beginnings of human existence, an order which demanded of its devotees a chastity beyond sexuality, a chastity uncompromising and unyielding. I was bound to the priesthood, married to it in a way I never felt married to any human. I was to be a good priest, a priest of the order of honorable practitioners of the healing arts. I did not sleep with patients.

In the subtlety of unintentioned eye movements, of unthought gestures, of non-verbal nuances, I let her know that while I felt a special kinship with her, enjoyed being with her, I was inexorably bound by the precepts of the priesthood.

CHAPTER 45

We are guardians of dreams. watchers over the future.

--a priest of the God of Fertility

Bellies in various stages of protrusion paraded past me. Checking routine obstetrical patients, an easy task once mastered, seemed formidable. Several misconceptions served as impediments to my education. First, I believed that babies were so fragile that they might crumble if one breathed upon them too hard. From this I reasoned that babies before birth were even more delicate and would shrivel if touched by any but the most skillful hands. I looked forward to the time when I would have to do a pre-natal examination myself with the utmost trepidation. After a minimal amount of small talk, a few standard questions were asked. The women then climbed awkwardly, always awkwardly, onto the exam table. I had been often struck by the lack of inhibition shown by my GYN patients. However, Pregnant women offended my highly developed sense of modesty more as they pulled their clothing up or down for the exam. I watched Steve Summerfield poke and prod belly after belly. He often called me to check the position of the baby, and ascertain whether it was engaged (that was when the baby's head was locked in the mother's pelvis just prior to delivery) or floating (that is still movable within the abdomen). Because of the time I had spent during a Christmas break in the office of a family physician who had a large OB patient load, I was able to catch on quickly. Summerfield, I could see, was impressed.

Though I was content to observe Summerfield for at least a week, my feelings were somewhat ambivalent. I was quickly becoming bored by the almost total lack of variation of the tummy checks. I was a doer, not a watcher. However, I was deathly afraid that I might miss some lesion and thus make both mother and child the victim of a major mishap. That I knew this fear to be unreasonable, did not lessen the hold of this belief on my psyche. However, Summerfield was an utter pragmatist. Such issues as these did not concern him. He knew that unlike most of my colleagues at my stage, I was both capable of and willing to work. The second day Summerfield gave me a room and a stack of charts. "You see these patients." He told me. He saw the unvoiced "but" in my eyes. "Don't worry," he soothed in a voice like honey, "everything will be alright." I remembered the two previous time he had told me this. I looked up and down the hall several times, fully expecting the immediate arrival of a major catastrophe. Only the yawning monotony of the dull semi-military routine could be seen. I called the first patient.

CHAPTER 46

We often try to find the nature of a thing by using words to define it. This is paradoxical as words, by their very nature, diminish the scope of that which they are used to describe and yet it is the nature of almost all things to expand as our knowledge of them deepens.

--the Heretic Priest on Truth

The delivery room was slow. I stretched legs too long for the worn pink scrub suit that stopped abruptly several inched above my ankles. The air was still. Neither of the two patients in the labor suite were near delivery. I looked at the intern, Norman Rollins, who spoke with several of the resident-priests at the far end of the long room, then, for the eighth time, at the same passage in the book I held across my thighs. A half-suppressed yawn escaped from my open mouth. The cadence of unstopped chatter at the end of the room was broken by a short burst of laughter. I turned to my book, a synopsis of obstetrics and gynecology. It contained eight hundred pages. Finishing one twenty-paged chapter on normal labor and delivery seemed more than I could accomplish. I tossed the small tome on a Masonite counter. It had been an hour since Norman had checked either patient. I rose, walking slowly through the long room to the corridor where the two women were in labor. A swash-swash-swash sound like that of an old washing machine could be heard as I approached the women's rooms. A breathless woman with blond hair looked up. Her belly protruded high above the padded surface of the stretcher. I looked at the monitor tape. I could see that she had just completed a contraction of medium intensity. I looked into the woman's-tired eyes.

"Hi! How're you doing there?" My mood was calm.

Fine." She smiled at me bravely.

"Good." I smiled. "Looks like your contractions are coming about every four minutes." I held the monitor tape in my hand as I read it. It did not appear as smooth or as free from artifact as those in the texts, but I was able to read it as a normal tracing. Footsteps sounded in the hallway.

"I told you that you shouldn't check the patients alone!" Norman, the intern, scolded me for only the third time that night. Though my patience with him had worn thin, I refrained from answering the boyish looking priest sharply. He meant that I was not to perform an internal exam without him present. It was also becoming abundantly clear that I was to do nothing while he examined the patients. He pointedly carried one examining glove. The woman looked at me puzzled as I had seen her initially and had spent far more time with her than the intern. Though my patience with Norman had worn thin, I refrained from answering him sharply. The patient needed all her courage for the ensuing delivery and did not need to witness the priest's in-fighting. I smiled to reassure her. I ignored the intern's comment.

"Time to check you again, " Rollins called out as he thrust his fingers deep into the woman.

"Oh, I hate this." The woman wrinkled her nose.

"Yeah." Rollins answered as he pushed his fingers further. Norman's face was a mask of concentration. "About seven to eight centimeters and . . . minus one station." He patted the woman's foot as he rose to leave.

"U-u-u," the patient sucked in her breath. "It's starting again." The monitor showed a contraction beginning. She breathed rapidly, too rapidly. "Breathe slow and easy." I encouraged the woman. "Breath slowly." I exhorted. "Try to relax." I stood watching the woman's face as she tried to follow my instructions. The undulations of the monitor which preceded those of the woman's body by several seconds showed that the contraction was diminishing. An easing inched across her sweat-studded brow. Her breathing took on a more regular pattern. Her face settled into a seriousness beyond her claim on years as she waited for the next wave of pain. I left the room quietly. My patients stared in front of her, hovering in the nether land between sleep and wakefulness.

As I passed from the far end of the long room to the place I had been sitting, Norman smiled at a comment of one of the priests. The grin seemed somehow to have lost its charm, its boyishness. There was an ice-laden edge to it which would have caused me to recoil had it not been for my own unvented anger.

Several times I made the journey across the long room, to the patient's room beyond. More often than not Norman would follow me and examine the patient. The woman's moans grew in intensity as the winds of a gathering storm. When there was no longer a silent space between them, the first cries of a human filled the air. I stood in the delivery room, draped in the robes of the God of Fertility, arms crossed--and empty.

I watched the delivery of the second ward of the priests of the God of Fertility before going to bed.

□ □ □ □ □

The morning was bright. I had had an uninterrupted night's sleep, something I had never experienced while on call. I hurried for morning report, fresh, but disappointed. The priest who had delivered the warning regarding the missed call stood before me, knotting a thick black tie. "You know, if you sleep all night, you won't get any deliveries." He pulled the cloth through the final loop as he spoke to me.

I squirmed under his dissecting gaze. The transparent blue of his eyes reminded me of the dye often used to mark uncut steel. His stare, like the steel was cold, hard, devoid of human warmth. I said nothing. He smiled, very much satisfied.

He turned to go. The sound of his boots took a short eternity to pass beyond the empty corridor. I waited only as long as it took him to go.

Morning report was near. I had to check my patients.

CHAPTER 47

Grant me equanimity that I may practice my craft successfully on all and pass judgment on none.

--prayer of a student-priest

Veteran's Day. The base's movements were slow compared to their normal brisk pace. Things felt somehow askelter. Thoughts of Grace drifted unpleasantly through my mind as ever felt but never seen phantoms. I followed Summerfield. He too had been unlucky enough to draw call of a holiday. We did not talk much. I sensed that the sluggishness of the day bore heavily upon him, too. I was assigned to Summerfield for the day. He was GYN triage officer. That meant that after making rounds on the GYN floor, he saw all the gynecology patients who arrived at the walk-in clinic.

The mid-morning saw the arrival of a sleepy sun and an only slightly more awake student-priest at a set of offices away from the main clinic area. I passed, with Summerfield, through several rooms painted in a drab naval gray-green. After looking in each of the rooms, Summerfield returned to the first suite. He stood in a large interviewing room which led to a number of exam rooms. He threw a magazine onto a gray-topped desk.

"I'll work out of these two rooms." The resident-priest indicated two rooms on his right. "That room over there and the interview room on the other side will be yours." It took several seconds for me to comprehend the words he had spoken. He smiled as my face slowly lit up. My own room. And an interview room to boot. I could hardly contain myself. I beamed with pride. "You know what you're doing now. Just discuss the case with me after you have examined them. O.K.?"

"O. K!" The day, gray and sluggish, became bright as if a shadow had been lifted from its face. Patients began to arrive at a steadily increasing rate which left both of us busy. Summerfield had planned a quiet day of reading and was annoyed by the steady flow. However, I was delighted for the experience as a first line care provider. My confidence in my clinical examination soared as I picked out subtle abnormalities which were confirmed by Summerfield.

The day wore on. A woman with half-combed, reddish-colored hair gathered into a single, uneven pony tail was shown into my office. She sat down across from me. She wore faded blue jeans and matching jacket over a printed blouse. Her clothing as well as her face showed several heavy deposits of dirt. I introduced myself. "Hi, I'm Miriam." She leaned confidentially toward me as she spoke. "I have this problem . . . " She related a tale of a vaginal discharge she had. She was not certain how long she had had it, only that it had been present for more than two weeks. As she spoke, it became clear that the cause of her infection might be a sexually transmitted disease. I explained this to her.

"I was kind of afraid of that, doc."

"Is it possible that you might have gotten it from your husband?"

"I don't know . . . doc, I was messing with this guy about six months ago, but we stopped when my old man came back about two months ago. You think I could have gotten it from him?"

"I don't think so."

"Could it be Jeff?" she muttered thoughtfully.

"Excuse me."

"Doc, I was thinking who it might be." She was quite

bemused and not the slightest bit embarrassed. "See there was this guy I was messing around with a couple of times about three weeks ago. I wondered if it could be him."

"It's possible."

"But you see," she leaned even further toward me so that her face was only a few inches from mine, "it could have been this other guy that I been messing with for the last two weeks."

I said nothing and prayed that my mask of indifference held until she left the room. It did.

CHAPTER 48

Life is the miracle. All else is common place.
--a street poet

James Jensen. An African priest, born in America. Skin smooth with neatly trimmed mustache. Ruggedly handsome. I came to know Jim the last two of my four weeks at Serra. It was from Jim that I learned obstetrics. Jim was a first-year priest of the God of Fertility. He was technically an intern but never treated as such. This was for several reasons. First, he had been a general medical officer in the Navy for several years and was thus considerably more competent and experienced than other interns who been in medical schools only months before. He had worked out a deal with his department whereby he did only six of the normal twelve month internship. Also, he out-ranked all the residents of the God of Fertility. Though I spent nights on-call with Jim, I passed my days with Larry Greenspan, the resident officially charged with teaching me obstetrics. I spent two weeks with Greenspan, a very suave resident-priest with straight black, always combed hair, and a very practiced smile. Greenspan thought the world of his good looks and spent every spare moment in front of a mirror admiring them. Ostensibly, my relationship with Greenspan was the same as that with Summerfield. Some of the time which I had saved Summerfield had been given back to me in the form of teaching. More often than not, however, when Greenspan and I finished clinic early because I saw patients, he would disappear and instruct me to do likewise. Several times when I showed him that I was determined to learn despite his reluctance to teach, he was forced both to further my education and give me begrudging respect. As I spent all my days with Greenspan, it was not until I was on-call at night that I got to know Jim Jensen. The first night we were on call together, I sat in my usual place at the far end of the main room of Labor and Delivery.

The conversation at the other end, as always, covered every topic but Medicine. Jim also sat at the far end of the room, bored. I leafed through a few pages. I placed the small tome on the counter.

□ □ □ □ □

After a time, Jim and I struck up a conversation. We talked for the better part of an hour.

"How many babies have you delivered?" Jim asked me.

"None." I tried hard to keep the disappointment from my face.

"How long you been here?"

"This is my third week."

He looked at me incredulously. "You haven't delivered any babies yet?"

"No."

"You know, you have to jump on those patients as soon as they hit the door."

"I've been following them."

"Then how come you haven't delivered any?"

"I can't check them without Norman. And once he checks them, he delivers them."

"Ma-a-an!" He looked at me knowingly for a time.

Before the nurse had completed her initial assessment of the next patient, Jim bounded from his chair. "Come on." He called to me. I followed close on his heels. As we passed the group of priests at the near end of the room, he called, "We're going to check this patient."

Norman looked up, smiled uncomfortably, said nothing. A twenty-eight year old woman was having her first child. Her husband stood at her side comforting her, calling words of encouragement. Through the course of the night, I checked her frequently with Jim. At the last possible moment, we took her into the delivery room. Jensen did one of the quickest scrubs I have ever seen, barely allowing the water to touch his skin. He rushed into the delivery room as I stood doing a more leisurely scrub.

"You better hurry, or you'll be too late." Jim yelled from within.

To hell with aseptic technique. I grabbed an unsterile paper towel and wrung the water off my hands. My hands still dripping, I put on a pair of gloves.

"Here. Control the head. Control the HEAD!"

"I got it. I got it."

"Alright, now. Watch it . . . go ahead and push." She pushed and screamed at the same time. She also managed to grab my arm. Her nails dug deep into my skin as the baby's head appeared. A guttural scream escaped from her lips. She released my arm. The rest of the baby came with relative ease. Though, I had been warned repeatedly about the force with which the tiny body could be propelled, I still nearly dropped the slippery, wet infant. I delivered the chord then helped Jensen with the episiotomy repair.

"It's a baby girl." Someone called. I had forgotten to look. We checked the baby again. She was fine. The mother was tearful, smiling. The father who stood at her side was imbued with pride.

"Thank you." She called. "I hope I wasn't too bad."

"No," I said as I rubbed my arm for the first of many times over the next several days, "you were just fine."

I watched Mrs. Fredericks being wheeled onto the ward. A warm glow like the aftermath of a loving kiss covered her face. I placed the robes of the priesthood, the green ones I wore over my pink ones, into the laundry bag.

"Boy!" I sighed. The book of obstetrics and gynecology was where I had left it on the counter top. I reached for it as I stretched my legs across a second chair. I heard my name called. The voice was angry.

I turned to look at Jim. "Yes?"

He came toward me with a small mound of records. "You got some paperwork to do."

"Oh!"

CHAPTER 49

Having once walked in the Sunshine of your smile,
I chase the setting sun.
--a student-priest and poet

Moonlight slither-slid over blue-black polished waves which rose and fell as the breath of a restive sea. In the quiet between tracts, during the planned pauses, I heard the thunder of the bay as a mild whisper. I sat at a corner table with Grace as she watched the dance floor, intently. I squeezed her hand lovingly, gently as I watched her face. I waited for a response. She was unaware of my presence or my touch. I shrugged my shoulders, disappointed. I then turned to the floor.

"Disco Inferno", a song from the Saturday Night Fever sound tract, quickened the pace. I felt my shoulders swaying involuntarily. The motion picture had marked America's sky-rocketing interest in the new art form, disco dancing. Inhibited by a near terminal case of shyness, I had ventured onto the dance floor only rarely during my adolescence. With the rise of disco, I was drawn to the dance floor many nights.

My feet tapped in time to the music. I pulled a reluctant Grace onto the floor. I reveled in the delirium of dance. Several more records found us on the floor. The driving drums and guitars dissolved into the soft "How Deep Is Your Love?"

As the Bee Gee's hummed, I pulled Grace closer, enjoying the nearness, the softness of her. We swayed gently in time to the music. I looked at my bride's face. Her eyes looked intently upon other couples as if something she sought lie there. She did not see me, did not see the affection, the love for her, in my eyes. I put my arm around her, trying to draw her closer, wishing with all my heart that I might accomplish by force of will what my love alone could not. She moved distractedly, unmindful of my presence. I turned again.

As I listened to the space between heart beats, an unanswered voice kept calling. I looked into the face of Grace and wondered how deep *was* our love.

CHAPTER 50

I am free of
neither pain nor blame in
our love.
--a student-priest and poet

Friday afternoon. Junipero Serra Park. Cars, hungry, aggressive beasts, sped past. Clinic and my responsibilities for the week were over. The park clock sounded, marking three-quarters past the hour of three o'clock. Things she had said had left more questions than answers. She had something to do, she had said, some business to take care of. I had played it cool. I had been disappointed too many times. The night on-call had been uneventful. Perhaps two deliveries the entire night. Morning report, something I always dreaded. passed quietly. She stated that she loved me still, that she still had unfinished business with Armstrong. She - intimated but stopped short of saying in so many words that she was through with him. I had told myself throughout the day that I should feel happy. Yet an ill-defined and unwanted foreboding gnawed at the back of my consciousness. Grace was to pick me up at four o'clock.

The clock struck five. Grace had not come. I did not know why but, I was not surprised. I brushed crushed green blades of grass from my pants. Across the street from where I stood, tired figures poured out of the clinics.

I turned to go home. After only a few steps I stopped. I needed my strength for the night to come, I thought. Again, I did not know why I felt this, only that I could not ignore the feeling.

I boarded a bus which took me to within two blocks of my home. The dreariness of my apartment was oppressive. I needed my car. At least if I could move, run, fly, I might be able to find a moment's respite. But my car was gone, I knew not where--and so was my wife. I felt as a caged beast, unable to find solace or freedom. My thoughts were drawn inexorably to Grace. Agitation reached a feverish peak as I pictured her with the never-seen, but ever-present Armstrong. I punched the buttons of Grace's number into my phone. There was no answer.

Driven by the rushing emptiness inside of me, an emptiness which I knew would only worsen no matter what I found at the end of my journey, closed the door of my apartment behind me.

CHAPTER 51

without you,
I cannot dream.
without you, there
is no Sun.
without you, I cannot dream.
--a poet of the House of Life

It was the time of day when, the ever-busy city finds peace within itself, the time of day when street lights stand like blue-white diamonds suspended over a land imbued with the red-golds, the fiery magentas of the setting sun. It was my most cherished time of day, a time when I often had my best thoughts.

It was Friday evening. The sun was leaving the sky. I wanted my wife, my one true love--I decided to settle for my car. I stood at the crest of one of the tallest hills in the city of canyons, a hill of gold and green. At the bottom of the hill lay the steep roadway which led to my wife's apartment. I stood watching the shimmer-shine of street lamps against the red sky.

As I mounted my bicycle, I imagined myself a brave and lonely warrior riding to a mission, a battle from which I might never return. Buttoning my coat slowly, deliberately, I smiled bitterly. My imaginings were altogether too close to reality. I lunged down the hill. I remember the azure and gold sky. I remember the white lights of cars at my side. I remember the wind blowing past my ears for too brief a time. I remember arriving at the foot of the hill which led to Grace's apartment. I remember the incline, which I attempted without dismounting only on the best of days. I remember ascending the steep grade quickly. I did not stop for rest.

I arrived at the crest of the hill panting for breath. What if Grace was not five-hundred miles away in Armstrong's home town, but right there with him in her apartment? It did not matter. I could not turn back. The quiet was disturbed only by the sounds of the distant highway and my own frantic breathing. A second, smaller entrance lay downhill from me.

My approach had been silent, swift, from the blind side of the complex. No one could come near or see me without me seeing them first. Good. I listened for every approaching car, surveying the occupants coldly, minutely. I looked over the parking lot, scrutinizing, in particular, two occupied cars. They represented no threat. It struck me that I was preparing for war, a very violent and desperate one. I mounted my bicycle. I pedaled rapidly as I searched each aisle for my car. It was not there. I skidded to a halt just before I reached Grace's door. There remained only the second entrance to the parking lot which lay near her apartment to be checked. I would walk by her door without stopping to ascertain who was within as I checked the final entrance.

As I passed her apartment, I found something unexpected. The door was ajar. Not knowing what to do, I stopped. I knocked. The door flew open. I peered into the semi-darkness. The three rooms of Grace's studio were each visible from the entrance. I stood at the doorway until, I was sure that no human form lurked in the corners. Slowly, one cautious step followed by another, I entered. I checked every inch, no one was there.

The disorganized array of clothes and furniture at first glance looked like the aftermath of a fight. No, no, I thought, not a fight, but hurried packing, the kind I had often seen Grace do.

Frustration and anger at Grace, Armstrong, the loss of my car, at a thousand wrong's perpetrated by her against me, great and petty welled within my mind. I thought to run, but I needed my car. I found the number of one of her friends, a colleague from law school, with whom she had frequent contact. I asked where was my car? He would not or could not tell me. I tried to think of other places she might leave it. My efforts were fruitless.

Anger mounted unabated. As I sat on her sofa, muscles taunt, my eyes came to rest on the multitude of letters she had left scattered about her living room. My thoughts turned to a time, a few months previously, when she had violated a great trust. She had entered my personal writings and read at random my most private thoughts. It had been a few months later, when *she* had confronted me angrily with what she had considered a personal affront to her that I had learned of her actions. She had demanded an explanation. I had given none. Instead, I would have demanded an apology had I thought that any words would lessen my sense of betrayal.

A scheme of retribution entered my brain. What better way to get hack at her than to read her letters? Thus, began one of the most sorrowful experiences of any life. The letters were many. There was a letter from her father which stated unequivocally that the suspicion which gnawed at my entrails was correct--she had long ago planned to divorce me. She had always denied this. Hurt began to replace anger, as I thought back to a mist-laden spring day when I had sat on a grass covered field trying with all the courage I had to get Grace to speak with me, to tell me what bothered her in our relationship, to open the clogged passages of communication. I had tried desperately to save a failed marriage. Grace had promised me that our separation was not permanent, that she only wanted time to get her head together. She knew as she had spoken these words that they had been untrue. I read further. There were a series of unfinished letters to Armstrong. All had been written over the previous several months and all except a few had a similar theme. The letters deplored his constant pleas for money. They described a relationship which was parasitic in nature. She told of a loan which she had given him but which he had never repaid. The money was the same sum I had loaned her when she had said she would be evicted. I had given up a much-needed vacation for this. She had likewise been unable to repay me.

There were plane tickets, boarding passes, chronicling several trips to Armstrong's hometown. There Was a love letter, more passionate than any I had ever received, more tender than any affection she had ever expressed for me. It described a night she and Armstrong had spent together in a romantic town overlooking the sea. The hurting was unbearable. Deep chasms of pain, like the molten fire of many volcanoes, welled within me, threatening to engulf me. Tears flowed freely for the first time in a long while as darkness enveloped the city of canyons, allowing me to hide my pain.

I was losing Grace. I had one last chance--call her. By methods which I still marvel at, I was able to track Armstrong through several moves and several towns. He had no phone, but received calls at the house of his sister-in-law who lived only twenty minutes away. I dialed the number. I left an urgent message for Grace to call me. That was not enough. I could fly there. But that would only create more problems. I sent a telegram, instead, asking her to call me. My last arrow spent, I returned to my empty apartment. I felt trapped. I needed to talk to someone, get away from Canon. I called Dr. Frank. His wife said that he was not in, that he would not be available for the next few days.

"Is this an emergency?" she asked, perhaps sensing the desperation I tried hard to hide.

"No, that's O.K. I can wait." I said mustering one last surge of control.

"I'll give him your message," she said politely with concern.

"Thank you." I said.

I called La Reina, the city I called home. I was lucky Samori was at home. I felt badly about calling him. He was struggling, I knew.

"Are you O.K., man?"

"I'm hanging on." I told him only that I was having trouble with Grace and that I needed to talk with him. "You want me to come get you?" He offered. Friends like Samori are hard to come by.

"No, I can make it up there."

"O.K., see you when you get here." Within two hours, I was in La Reina.

CHAPTER 52

Love and time have healed more wounds than priests.
--the Heretic-Priest

I'll **be home in** a while, Mom." My mother's face with its smiling cheeks, the cheeks I loved in any woman, the cheeks which were the hallmark of her progeny, was saddened. She could see that her youngest son, her doctor son, was shaken. She knew that Grace and I had separated. She did not know what had brought her son home. "You take care of yourself, now," she called.

"Bye, Mom." I called as I reached the final stair of the painted red brick porch. The evening was overcast and cold. I enjoyed the walk, though I was impatient to arrive at my destination. I skirted traffic on the large avenue, then turned quickly into an anonymous, but familiar, side street.

The passage way which led to the wood frame house ran on the edge of the property. My steps were guided more by memory than the light of the fading dusk. "Hello." I called. As I approached, a heavy wooden door opened.

"What's happening?" Samori stood in the doorway.

"What's happening?" I answered. Samori opened the screen door. I entered, glad to feel the warmth of the house as it rushed at me. My eyes fell upon familiar furniture, stone fire place, stereo. We sat in a nook in the living room. For a while we made s mall talk.

"Well. what 's all this that ' s been happening. man?"

“I don 't know." I had not spoken to Samori in some months about Grace and I. brought him up to date on all the events of the last few months and the last weekend.

We then spoke of many things, of my loves, his loves, of loves gone wrong of fidelity, infidelity, of the insanity and usefulness of both. We spoke of places, people, things for many hours. We spoke of our childhood and adolescence. Time flowed like warm water in a gentle whirlpool. taking us in ever higher spirals, and finally setting us down softly
where we had begun. I was left with my inner peace restored.

Thanks. said as e I 1eft.

"Hey, man you 're my brother."

Thank you anyway."

It was a quick walk home.

CHAPTER 53

I hide within the shadows of a love which knows not love. I
hide within the shadows of a growing fear, afraid to face
the loneliness that envelopes me.

--confession of a student-priest

Sunday morning. The City of Canyons. I awoke to yellow-gray rays of sun settling tentatively upon a forest green carpet. I lay still several minutes before I rose, afraid that even the slightest movement might disrupt my fragile equanimity. The peace of a mid-night ride to Canon and an undisturbed slumber held as I pushed my body to the edge of the bed. I had to face the morning. I thought briefly of Grace., of the futility of denying that she was with Armstrong. I did not need such thoughts. What I needed was an itinerary, a structure on which to hang the disjointed fragments of my day. I decided upon a leisurely hot bath to occupy my morning followed by an equally leisure bike ride to Serra Park.

□ □ □ □

A high-pitched whistling sounded intermittently as I spun the red three-speed bicycle. I re-adjusted the wheel. The high-pitched noise stopped. I returned the bike to its upright position.

The phone rang. Perhaps it was Grace. No, that was unlikely. I doubted that Grace would contact me before she got home. I did not expect her until late in the evening. It was probably a wrong number or a salesperson.

"Hello" I answered the phone

"Hello, sweetheart. What 's the matter?" The voice was full of concern several seconds passed before I was able to accept the reality. It was Grace!

"I'm O.K.". I answered. Joy and elation overcame me but quickly turned to pain and disappointment as I anticipated the answer to the question I had to ask.

Where was she?

"I'm at home. I read your note. Are you O.K.?" Grace spoke of the note I had left asking her to call. me when she arrived.

"I missed you. I need to talk to you." I told her.

"I missed you, too." she spoke with anticipation. "I'm coming right over. Bye." She hung up the phone.

I met her on the steps.

Grace arrived within five minutes.

We shared a warm and intimate embrace.

I spoke earnestly of the love I had, that I hoped that she yet shared

"I wish you had told me all this before," she cooed.

We spoke a while longer. I told her of the calls I had made

"You did *WHAT*?" Fire flashed in her eyes. The Ann of anger and bitterness, the one I had seen all too often was with me again. "You stupid . . ." she did not finish. "I'll be god damned!!" She called out. "I'll be god damned!!" She shouted " Do you know what you did?" She paused only a second.

I had called to say that I wanted and loved her, I told her.

"I'll be god damned." She tossed my explanation, my plea for understanding, for forbearance aside as insignificant, irrelevant. She continued berating me, using every curse word, every invective she knew. A myriad of emotions flooded my mind. Foremost among these was anger and fear. Anger at the acute injustice of her attack and fear that after coming so close to regaining my lost bride, I was losing her again--forever. As I could say nothing to make her want to stay, I chose to say nothing.

Three hours later, her anger finally spent, she stopped. She asked could she use the phone. I told her she could.

She ran the water for a bath as she pulled the phone into the bathroom. Her voice rose in hoarse whispers, then raucous laughter. I sat on the couch, staring at the carpet.

Silence pointed a mocking, accusing finger at me. I went into the bedroom where I kept my records. I could make out Grace's words clearly. I did not wish to hear them. I turned on the record player. Still I heard her clearly.

"Yeah, man. I don't know where he got the numbers from, but that fool called *everybody*." There was a short pause followed by a prolonged peal of ribald laughter. She continued her deprecations. I could take no more hurt.

The screen door slammed behind me as I stepped into the chilled evening air. Twilight, the time of change, was upon the magenta and gold sky.

□ □ □ □

Weeks passed as I tried to erase the events of that evening from my memory, as I tried to suppress a smoldering rage. I was successful at neither task. Moreover, an unrelenting fear grew within me because, for the first time since I had known Grace, I could not forgive.

CHAPTER 54

Heresy is the name we sometimes give to that part of us which subscribes to higher values.

--the Heretic Priest

Though I had been to almost every other hospital connected with the medical school, I had never been to St. Mary's. It stood on the edge of a steep gorge, overlooking the center of the city of canyons. High atop its tall beige walls stood a large white cross, a beacon to those sick and in need of solace. People in many shades of white, green, or blue uniforms traversed long crisply painted driveways quickly, quietly, orderly. The careless, reckless gregariousness seen in the young warrior priests at the U and the V.A. was not seen at St. Mary's. Instead a near-silent simplicity reigned where each had his or her place and titles, not loudness, were the only keys which opened doors. I traveled along the sidewalk to the main entrance. Only the sound of my footsteps disturbed the quietude. I placed my black bag in my left hand so that I could make final adjustments to my clothing as I neared the doorway. Drawing my body erect, I stepped forward boldly. The automatic door opened as I reached out to touch it. I tried to regain my balance and self-confidence as I nearly stumbled into an elderly couple. I was half-way down the corridor before I realized that the guard, whom I fully expected to challenge me when I had entered the building, had only nodded and smiled as I had passed. For several seconds, I stood at the junction of two large hallways wondering which of three banks of elevator I should take. After several seconds, the guard approached me.

"Can I help you, doctor?" Doctor? Though I wore my white coat. My name tag clearly lacked those all-important letters, M.D. His face pink and clean-shaven, searched mine earnestly. I stood as tall as I could, at least three inches taller than my actual height.

"Can you direct me to the pediatric ward?"

"Sure. You go down this corridor."

"Uh-huh."

"See those elevators to the left there?"

"Yes."

"Take those to the fifth floor."

"You want to go to the nursery or the place for the bigger kids?"

"Just the regular ward will be fine."

"O.K. When you get off the elevator, make a left then a sharp right. That'll put you right there on the pediatric floor." He repeated the directions to me. I thanked him.

The elevator deposited me at the pediatric floor. I stood uncertainly for a moment. A slightly obese woman sat behind a desk writing.

"May I help you?" Both her demeanor and tone were polite.

"I'm looking for the pediatric house staff."

"They usually meet in the back room about this time. "She indicated a room behind the nurse's station. "I don't think they're there yet, though."

I thanked her then walked into a large room behind the front desk. My eyes fell upon a brown-skinned woman whose hair was hurriedly combed in an uneven Afro. Though it was the first time I had ever seen her I knew immediately that she was Sarah, the never-seen, but often spoken of priest of the God of Children. She was one of a very few student-priests of African descent who had continued their residency at Canon. I had heard much about her. In the meetings of the Semi-secret Society, it was said that she lived with a male of

European descent and shunned all things and people African. From these and other things I had heard of her, I foresaw a difficult two weeks, probably more difficult than the previous four weeks spent with the sanguine priests of the God of Fertility.

I studied the short, strongly built woman as she churned through the pages of a chart. She had an almost palpable presence, an unquestionable authority about her. I watched her, saying nothing for the space of half a minute.

"So, you're one of the new medical students." She spoke to me. She raised her head only as she spoke the last word.

"Yes." I answered, startled. I had not known that she was aware of my presence. I said my name.

"Hello, George." Her tone was mockingly condescending.

"I'm Sarah Lord." She looked me full in the face. "I'm chief resident." Her statement had been unnecessary. It was clear that she was in charge.

"Hi. Pleased to meet you." I smiled.

She cast a reserved, but genuine smile my way. Her elbow rested on the counter as she returned to the chart.

"Where are your fellows?"

"They're on their way inside the building. In fact, they should be here already." Rich and Pat had been looking for a parking space as I arrived. Sarah said nothing.

"Where are the other house staff?"

"Late." Annoyance filled her voice. "They're always late." I said nothing further as I did not wish to become the target of her unspent wrath. We stood for a few moments as I rummaged through the three objects in my black bag as if I were looking for something I had not already found.

A group of boisterous voices approached. I recognized that of Francisco who liked to be called Frank. He led a band of first-year priests of the Child God. As the interns neared the elevator, the doors opened. My classmates exited in a mood as jovial as that of the child priests. The two groups exchanged warm greetings. The priests and medical students continued toward the chief resident.

"Hi, Sarah." Frank spoke to the priest of the Child God.

“God morning!" Irritation permeated her voice. "Let's start."

"But I haven't finished my breakfast yet." Frank called in mock protest as he chewed a bagel laden with half a cup of cream cheese. Sarah cast a stern glance at the intern as she pushed the chart rack to the middle of the floor.

"Alright, alright." Frank conceded. He held the bagel firmly in his mouth as he searched for a chart. thin cloud of crumbs was airborne as he whipped though several pages. ". . . O.K., here we go." Pieces of cream cheese fell from his mustache. Michael's Conway. Let's see" He scanned the last page of writing. "His white count is down to eight thousand with six bands." Frank closed the book. "He is now afebrile times thirty-six hours."

"Plan?" John Peters, an intern, nudged Francisco.

"Huh"?

"What are you going to do with him?"

"Oh, yeah. Plan is to send him home today on oral penicillin for a week.

Sarah spoke to the intern. "Maybe you can give a brief history for the medical students."

"Sure. Michael is a six year old boy in his seventh hospital day who was being treated for right lower lobe pneumonia with I.V. penicillin. He is now on oral penicillin 250 milligrams q.i.d."

"Follow-up?" Sarah spoke again. "He's going to be followed by his private medical doctor." "Good. Don't forget to notify the parents."

"I'll do that right after rounds."

"Next? Room 507."

Each of us waited. We students, in our clean white coats, striking what each of us felt was his best academic pose, each hoping he would not be called upon to answer a question. All the house staff except John stood at bored attention, looking at some indeterminate point between the ground and their knees. John's attention seemed transfixed by the intricacies of the traffic several floors below.

"Next!" Sarah called impatiently.

The priests shifted restlessly. Frank brought his elbow into John's side. "Five-O-Seven. That's you." Frank's voice was a loud whisper.

"That's me? . . .Oh yeah, that *is* mine."

"What's the matter with you guys today?" Sarah chided the priests.

A business-like mood settled over the priests. Rounds continued at a slow, deliberate pace. A few rooms later we were mat by a tall tanned priest with auburn hair. Sanford Hamilton had the facial features and physique of a model in an advertisement for beach front vacations. His khaki slacks and sandals made it seem that the dress shirt and white coat he wore were only reluctant concessions to convention and his position of resident priest. He had been taking care of a problem. As second in command, Sanford was responsible for day to day details. He took the whip from Sarah. The interns moved. Rounds were interesting at St. Mary's. There was no rushing between rooms at commercials in order to catch the next television segment as there had been at the U. Instead, conversation and attention was absorbed in patient care. Medical students were not treated as useless appendages. We were brought into rounds as active participants. We were challenged, chided, involved. All these were due in large part to Sarah. My respect and affection for her grew daily as I was exposed to not only an outstanding teacher, but an excellent physician and warm human being. "She really knows her stuff, doesn't she?" Pat Stein confided in me. "Yes, she does." I beamed with pride

I marveled that my opinion of this diminutive woman changed so radically in so short a time. I passed a very pleasant two weeks under the tutelage of the chief resident of the God of Children.

CHAPTER 55

The chronically ill pediatric patient is inflicted with a disease he/she can neither comprehend nor control. More often than not one parent (usually the father) has deserted them. Also, their illness curtails their activities and seriously hampers normal development. Small wonder he/she is a very angry individual and particularly difficult to manage.

--lectures, House of the Child God

M**iguel Baron,** a tall, angular eleven year old male, in no acute distress, presented in diabetic ketoacidosis.

"He did not take his insulin for two days." An old woman spoke plaintively to Sanford Hamilton, the first-year pediatric resident. Thick, stiff legs supported the woman's large chest and protuberant belly. "Yeah."' He said for lack of something else to say. He had already heard the history and initiated treatment. The only thing remaining was to wait and re-evaluate the boy in a few hours. "Do you think he's very sick?" The woman spoke in a Spanish accent. "Yeah, he's sick." Sanford said, looking at the boy. Miguel, whose eyes did not leave the television set, was visibly concerned with Sanford's words. "But he'll be alright." The priest added.

"You think so?" the old woman asked. Her eyes, brown and shining with moisture, showed redness.

"Oh, sure," he assured her.

The woman, the boy's paternal grand-mother moved closer to the boy's bed. Her face held an expression of helpless concern. The boy looked not at her, but at the television as he sat on the bed. Sanford moved to leave.

"Doctor?" The woman said the word as it was pronounced in Spanish, with the accent on the last syllable. Sanford turned. "There is a doctor who speaks Spanish. Do you know where he is?"

"I speak Spanish." Rodger told the woman.

"Oh!" The woman answered with surprise. That Sanford spoke Spanish did not correspond to the image I had of him.

What's wrong with him, why is he so sick? the woman asked in Spanish.

Sanford answered in Spanish fluent and grammatical. He told her that the I.V. was needed to give Miguel insulin so that his blood sugar could be brought under control. Also, that Miguel might be in the hospital a few days to accomplish this task.

The old woman thanked the resident-priest earnestly. Sanford left the room. The woman stood before the boy, hands on hips, with the same concerned expression, as she admonished him in Spanish. Why did you do this? There was great tenderness in her scolding. Didn't you know it would make you sick? The boy lowered his dark brown eyes. "Parquet?" Why? she asked.

I left silently.

CHAPTER 56

Experience is unquestionably the greatest teacher. However, the advancement of humankind would be immeasurably furthered by the development of another, equally effective method.

--a priest of the God of Life

Floating. I was floating, drifting without control. I was trying to fasten on to something, anything solid. It was in the formless area between cognitive and intuitive knowledge, that area called judgment, that I grappled with the problem of our new charge. Even the old priests, veterans of many wars, were baffled. It was a judgment call. I had no judgment. I had only a beautiful little girl with a pain in her hip. Did she have a true bacterial infection, which needed immediate surgical drainage or was she simply manifesting an unusual presentation of a virus?

Inuncía spent hours at a time earnestly arranging her dolls, placing them, at the edge of her window, in neat, happy rows. As I watched Inuncía play, it was difficult to imagine that her eight year old body harbored a disease which could leave her crippled for life. It was difficult to believe that she was ill at all. Yet the pain in her hip as we examined her was undeniable. The priests of the Child God pondered the pain of the little girl. They pondered the cause of her continued low-grade fever, the small, but persistent elevation of both her white count and sed rate. Were these simply signs of a virus as might cause a cold, or were they the signs of an insidiously growing infection? A priest of the God of the Knife pondered these same questions by night. Several times I saw him as I left late or was on-call. Often, in worried whispers, we spoke of our concern for our young charge. Many times, he asked my opinion earnestly, watching my face as I spoke. Each time I admitted that I, and the priests of the Child God, were as baffled as he.

In the end, the priests did not have an answer, nor did I find one in any of the sacred texts. All agreed only that the answer to Inuncía's hip lay in judgment, judgment based on experience, judgment based on seeing a hundred cases like this one, judgment which I, a fledgling student-priest of the House of Life, did not have.

During quiet moments at home and as I walked the wards of the God of Children, I grappled with the questions of the little girl, her painful hip, and judgment.

CHAPTER 57

As I am priest, I am human.
--a priest of the House of Life

Grace was in trouble again. She had found an eviction notice hanging on her door, *again*. Her rent was three months behind, *again*. She had no way to pay it. What could she do, she asked me? I had no money. How could I help her? My mind went back to a time some eleven months before when she had been in similar circumstances. Then, however, I had not known if I could survive without Grace. The ensuing year had been a crucial one for me. I had arrived at the edge of the realization that I could survive without Grace.

Now Grace was in trouble--again. She needed a place to stay--again. I could offer her my home or deny her plea for help. I still wanted her; I knew. I also knew that desperation was no longer my master. I could accept or reject any offer. Still, Grace needed help and I loved her. I knew there was but one choice I could make and still consider myself a decent person. I promised myself that I would not make a decision for a week, but in the space of a faltering heart beat, the promise was nullified when Grace called once again. I offered her my home. She accepted.

CHAPTER 58

The God of Internal Medicine has many faces. One is that of a large voracious insect with long, needle-sharp sucking mouth parts. In this aspect, it is both menacing and sanguine. The surgeons call the priests of Internal Medicine, fleas after the insect form of the internists' deity.

--historical notes of the Priesthood

Life is a series of crises. There is the crisis of birth followed by the crises of adolescence, adulthood, middle-age. The training of the priests of the House of Life is itself a crisis filled with smaller crises. One of these is the third year. Within the third year there is generally one clerkship which stands head and shoulders above the others in difficulty. At most medical schools this clerkship is surgery. At Canon, it was Medicine 1. Medicine 1, the name whispered with unreasoned dread and fear. Medicine 1 with its somber, never smiling priests. Medicine 1, the crisis of the third year. "You're taking medicine next quarter, aren't you?" Tim's normally soft voice seemed even softer. I was distracted. I focused upon his question.

"Yes." I answered. But what did that have to do with anything? "Louis and I are taking it next quarter, too." Tim continued, stretching his long frame as he smoked. As I watched him take a puff, then extend a glowing cigarette what seemed like a quarter of a mile to the far reach of his arms, I was reminded of the special name Grace and I had for Tim. We called him "that long boy" as much for his childish innocence as his unusual height. I smiled a little to myself. I was fully focused on Tim, but I did not follow his train of thought. Vaguely I remembered that after the lottery which had been held in the spring, I had found that Tim, Louis, and I would all take Medicine in the winter quarter. During the struggle of first Surgery, then Peds/OB-GYN I had lost track of my fellows.

Tim continued. "Louis and I thought it would be good if we stuck together during this. That way we could help each other out." Two weeks previously I had received a letter which asked the students taking Medicine 1 the coming quarter to choose groups of three or four students depending on whether they started at the V.A. or at the University Hospital. "You mean the three of us would be in the same group?" I asked.

Tim searched my face. "Yeah."

"Sounds good to me."

"Good." Tim spewed a stream of gray white air across the room, away from me. "I already turned our names in." Footsteps sounded distantly behind us. "Who's the fourth member of our group?"

"Reggie Rand." A question was on my face. "You know Reggie, don't you.?"

"No, I don't think I do."

“He's a good guy."

"Oh."

□ □ □ □

Cap, short for Captain, sat across from me. He was a student priest of African descent who had entered with me. Unlike me, however, he was in the fourth year class.

"You're doing WHAT?!!!" His tone was accusing, argumentative. It piqued an angry chord in me.

"We're taking medicine together." I repeated slowly, deliberately as if speaking to a dull child.

"The three of you are going to be on the same team?" Cap glared across the table.

"Yes." I answered annoyed. I had said it plainly enough already. Cap viciously stuffed the remnants of a bologna sandwich into his mouth. The student-priest's cheeks were stuffed like that of a small squirrel. He chewed quickly.

"You must be crazy!" He spat out. His tone intimated that this was his final decree, his ultimate judgment of Tim, Louis, and I, our plans. I watched him minutely for several seconds. My eyes fell upon his retreating hairline, his stuffed jowls. I thought of several hurtful things I knew and a thousand more I had surmised or suspected. I thought of calculated and cruel ways to say them, then stopped. Once the battle was begun, I knew I could not stop. I did not wish to draw psychic blood.

"I've got work to do." I said as I rose. It was not a battle worth fighting, I told myself as I struggled for control. "Later." "Bye." He said curtly. Tension filled the air. My feet sounded a gallop down the hallway.

Why had Cap's comment angered me so? Oh, who cares? I really did have work to do. I did not have time to fight with him. Cap's sentiments, I found, were shared by many student-priests. Whenever I said that we were teaming up together, the first question was always the same--are you crazy? The cloud of a lingering doubt stayed in my mind—*was I*? I argued with myself. Students of European descent had always teamed up together, gaining support from their friends. Why not us? I tried to convince myself that we were not headed for disaster.

Are you crazy? The words kept echoing in my brain. *Were we?*

In the weeks before the beginning of the winter quarter, the quarter of Medicine 1, doubt weighed heavily upon my mind.

CHAPTER 59

As waves wash out to sea, I say I must go,
and as they return headlong to the shore,
morning will find me in your arms.

--Love's Rhapsody and Waning[1]

(A poem by George Saunders)

Recall a time soft and warm, gentle and mist-laden. Recall a quiet, joyful time when my twice lost love was back at my side. Recall a time when I basked in the brownness of her eyes, rode to the sky on the wings of her touch, felt no greater happiness than the warmth in her arms. There passed a time idyllic and peaceful, one of the happiest in my life, when we ate, made love, fought, made love, made love, made love. As we made love, my eyes overflowed and I cried. I cried for all the nights that I was alone when I had not wanted to be alone, all the nights I had wanted my love. I cried for a thousand hurts given and suffered, for a marriage which was impossible to live with or without. I cried for Grace, for me, for the children we would never share, for the impossibility of our relationship enduring, for its undeniable endurance. I cried for many things--for failures large and small, untouchable across time, for hopes long nurtured and long lost

Yet time poured rich and free like honey from a wide-mouthed jar as we bathed in a sea of warmth and affection. We found time only for making love and each act of love was ecstasy and fulfillment. Thus, passed a time rich, beautiful, and happy beyond compare.

CHAPTER 60

Honor you your priests!

-instructions to the students-priests entering the House of the God of Internal Medicine.

Christmas break ended and with it the bliss-filled time of Grace and George. Freshly arrayed in the garb and tools of the priesthood, I kissed my bride good-bye one January morning. My kiss was like ice for already I had joined the battle of the dreaded Medicine 1. The visions in my eyes were those of silent battles punctuated by the amount of blood that could be let before one's adversary screamed, conflicts perpetuated by the fearful against the unknowing. Grace looked at me oddly for the space of a second. She said nothing, only held me as I stood in the doorway. She had seen her warrior-spouse steeled for battle before. She did the most that she or anyone else could have done.

Fortified with an extra touch of her love, I braved the gray dawn.

□ □ □ □

Cars, trucks, vans passed noisily in the Monday morning rush. Though I walked slowly, I was at the University Hospital, "the U." as it was called by the staff who worked there, long before I was ready. I decided to go to the main entrance, on the far side of the hospital, delaying the moment when I would have to begin my new clerkship. I paused in front of the brown blandness of the hospital, resisting the forces pulling me within. I stood for a long minute, trying not to appear that I was hesitating as several of my classmates passed. The appointed hour drew nearer. I knew no amount of time could dispel the dread which clung to my body tenaciously, like an unsatisfied lover. Standing there. In front of the U. only made things worse. Calling once again upon the stone man within me to move forward, I pushed through the double doors, ploughed into the elevator like a man jumping from an unavoidable cliff. Both Louis and Tim were already in the elevator. The three of us made nervous small talk as the car neared the top of the building. We exited at the 9th floor. The 9 West team, our team, was rounding. Behind a two-tiered rack on which all the charts were held, stood a short thin man with brown curls arrayed wildly about his head. Beside him stood a crystal blue eyed, thickly built man. His blond, conservatively cropped hair was noticeably lighter than his darker mustache. Speaking clearly, crisply, as we approached, in an argumentative tone was a harried appearing woman. Her barely combed hair, the color of burnished gold, was cut short on all sides and hung tamely over her head. Shiny and new, we stopped before the three priests. "Hi!" -Tim offered a warm but tentative greeting. Louis and I smiled. The priests looked directly at us, then shared between themselves a knowing, askance look. Without so much as a nod to acknowledge our existence or greeting, the priests, with whom we were to spend almost all our waking hours for the next - six weeks, continued rounds.

CHAPTER 61

Succor your priests in times of need.
--a priest's prayer

Tim's voice was streaked with fear as he began. Each of the four student priests had been repeatedly criticized for his formal presentation of cases. Some criticisms were expected. They were part of the learning process. The three remaining student-priests sat sullenly, uneasily as Ron moved with over-whelming trepidation into the first few lines of his prepared speech. Our eyes flashed fire as the priests passed ridiculing smiles between themselves. We waited for the all too familiar scenario of 9-West attending rounds to play itself through. We waited, with barely contained anger, for the first interruption which would signal the beginning of Tim's humiliation. Schnauzer led the attack. "What was the 'crit?" Tim stumbled, then answered. More questions followed. Tim tried to continue. Further interruptions. Tim was shaken further. His presentation began to resemble a hodge podge of unrelated information. Louis, Reggie, and I exchanged angry glances. Schnauzer delivered the final blow. He gave an impatient one-minute capsule summary from the beginning as if the
student-priest had said nothing. Tim's expression was one of abject defeat.

Tim left the room to get the chart so that the attending -priest, Donald, could sign it. "Don't they teach you guys basic stuff before you get on the wards? He should at least be able to do a physical." Donald, the veteran of proudly held liberal convictions, looked at the student-priests for a reply. I glared at the wall as a string of expletives went through my mind.

Tim returned.

Each of the student-priests had been through the same ordeal with the same result. As a group we had spoken with Schnauzer, Spears, and North. We had asked simply not be bombarded with unwarranted interruptions. We had explained that no one could present adequately under the conditions we faced daily. We had extracted a promise from the priests to allow us to tell our cases without unnecessary interruptions. The promise was broken with the very next presentation.

It was not until nearly the end of our stay at the U. that we struck upon a strategy that ended the constant harangues and humiliation. We became as nasty as our house staff. Every uncalled-for interruption or request for information outside of the formalized order of presentation was answered with a tersely uttered retort.

Soon thereafter, we were commended for our much-improved presentations.

CHAPTER 62

The stages of failure of almost every organ, has an uncanny uniformity which varies little with disease process.

--academy lectures, pathology course

"Joyce **McNair's** back in. Your team has her." A student-priest with nervous mannerisms and a sharply cropped mustache called to me in passing. He said the name as if it were one I should recognize. I did not. As I was not up for the next admission, my interest in the patient was detached.

"She did pretty good this time. She hasn't been in in a while," the student intimated to me.

"Yeah? How long?" I asked.

"Two months."

I was glad she would not be mine.

She advanced slowly through the corridor, an adored queen, home after a long journey. She arrived on 9-West, atop a stately stretcher, wearing a fresh hospital gown and two deeply cleft dimples.

"Hi!" Tim stopped before the returning queen. His voice was warm and empathetic. Tim told Joyce his name. "I'm the medical student who will be following you." He told her as he clasped the Masonite clip board which rested at his waist.

"Hi!" Joyce giggled. Her face beamed. She had developed an immediate crush on my tall and handsome classmate. Watching the two of them together, notwithstanding that Tim did not share his charge's feelings, was as watching two children at play.

CHAPTER 63

At its worst, lupus is a relentless adversary which attacks virtually every organ system, leaving none unscathed.

--academy lectures, lupus--
disease of a thousand faces

F**ever. What was** the source of the fever? For the second night running Joyce McNair had spiked a fever. With each peak of her temperature curve came a seizure.

Schnauzer examined Joyce again. The intern examined the patient again. Ron examined her again. He was joined by his three fellow student-priests. Each of us hoped to uncover some overlooked detail and thereby reveal the source of Joyce's fever. We found no answers. Consultants from virtually every medical sub-specialty made rounds on an almost hourly basis. Each pondered long and diligently over our charge. Each wrote long wordy passages. Each left us without answers. After several days, a shadow which would have been passed off as normal on any other patient, appeared on Joyce's chest x-ray. It grew, as if in answer to our prayers, into a definite infiltrate. The 9-West team breathed a collective sigh of relief. Joyce's face, the color of sun-bleached palms, kept its perennial smile throughout all.

The infiltrate was but the beginning of the teaching we received from our pleasant charge with the nine-volume chart.

CHAPTER 64

If our calling, our Gods, our God, is the same, then does our conflict not demean us all?

--The Semi-Secret Question

Both internship and the third year are very special times when the frightened and vulnerable intern or clerk (medical student) leans heavily on the calm, solid figure of the resident-priest. Often a bond is formed which is looked upon fondly in ensuing years. At the very least there is lingering awe of one who has done it all, seen it all, learned it all and not been overwhelmed. I am sure that a small bit of these feelings color my remembrances of Frank Schnauzer, my first resident in the House of the God of Internal Medicine.

Hair which reminded me of coiled flaxen serpents played above thick glasses and steel wire-rimmed blue eyes. His facial expression was always an unlikely mixture of unrestrained bemusement and stern severity. I often wondered did Frank have a private joke that he did not wish to share with the rest of us. The resident-priest was aloof,
imperturbable, and lukewarm to everyone. He was also unquestionably one of the brightest residents I have ever known. Under Frank were two interns, Jay North (Jay the Slow as he was

called by me) and Bonita Spears (her name varied with each student priest according to his proficiency in profanity). Jay was of thick-bodied, well-muscled Nordic stock. His painfully slow, nasal speech belied the substantive nature of what he said and the stellar quality of his work.

Bonita's hurriedly combed hair was worn always in a poorly pinned bun, giving her the appearance of one perennially harassed. Her hair, angular features, and terse, unhappy eyes, the color of a clouded blue sky, gave her an air of misery matched only by that which she meted out to those under her. A cold pragmatist, she managed the labors of her two student priests with exacting efficiency. Our daily tasks were given out each morning, quickly, briskly, with a minimum of conversation and were expected to be carried out in the same manner. For our diligence, obedience, slave-like service, Louis and I, the students under Spears, were fed a parsimoniously portioned diet of crumbs from the feast of knowledge of the House of the God of Internal Medicine.

On our first day on 9-West, the student-priests were required to know all the old patients as well as any new admissions. It was not an easy task to digest the volumes of charts of patients who had been on the wards for weeks as well as write up new admissions. I bore the burden silently and only slightly begrudgingly. It was no more than was expected of the students of other teams, I thought. However, I found that this was not the case. As I commiserated with other students-priests over the trials of third year clinical clerks, amazement filled their eyes. No such burden was placed upon the students of any other team. It was but the first of many ways in which the student-priests of 9-West were subjected to a very *special* treatment.

CHAPTER 65

I do not know what Death is. I know only that I fear it.

--a student-priest of the House of Life

My **first encounter with** Death's approach was in the beginning of my tour in the House of Internal Medicine, when I was but a frightened fledgling of the terrible wards. Bones and sagging flesh were wrapped in a dried, plastic sack-like covering'. Thin lips, which circled a toothless mouth, were seemingly drawn into his lungs with each breath. The small, wasted-appearing man stared vacantly through dull, glossed eyes. He barely moved as he was wheeled into his room. I carried a fresh blood sample to the clerk's desk. I paid little attention to the man on the stretcher.

Tiredness was beginning to set in. It was 10 P.M. My work was only half done. Two nurses behind me spoke as I labeled the sample. "Is that Mr. Hale?"

"Yes."

"What's he have?"

"Lung cancer." The reply was casual, matter-of-fact. "He's here for terminal care." Terminal care meant that the man had come to die.

I took the blood to the lab. It had cost both the patient and me too much to allow it to be lost on the way.

□ □ □ □

The next morning a shriveled figure lay on the bed, barely able to meet the demands of quiet breathing. My mind went back to the night before. Yes, this was the man dying of lung cancer. We mumbled a few words at each bed, the resident-priest approving or modifying the days plans.

We approached the man's bed, the intern spoke. "How are you today, Mr. Hale?" There was no response. The man looked at the ceiling as if we were not there.

"I don't think he heard you." someone said.

The resident spoke loudly. "Mr. Hale?" The man moved a little. "Mr. Hale?" The resident shouted louder. Mr. Hale looked toward the resident. "Are you hurting anywhere?" The man shook his head, no. "O.K. then, Mr. Hale." The priests moved away slowly.

I lagged behind the rest of the team. I had often heard nurses, and less seldom priests, say that they could discern the dying patient by a certain never described look. I wondered was this so. Though Mr. Hale barely looked alive, I could find no telltale signs that Death was about to descend. The mark of Death was not in his strangely smooth and shining skin, nor was it in the flaccid flesh that sagged from his threadbare bones. I could discern it nowhere.

Mr. Hale's face reminded me of the unfortunate lover of a goddess of ancient Greece who had cruelly been granted immortality, but not eternal youth. After many years, he had become a grasshopper to roam the earth no longer human.

As I continued to look at our charge's face, I saw much to pity but nothing of the specter Death. I looked at him once again, stepping back with both my mind and my body. It was then that I saw lines much more delicate than the lines of his face. What I saw was something of this world, yet not of it. It was the spirit, perhaps the skeleton of the soul of our unfortunate charge. It was tired and gnawed as if some ravenous and cowardly beast had bitten pieces of it while our charge yet lived.

Later that night, the animal, Death, gathered Mr. Hale in its jaws and carried him, with little ceremony, to his grave.

CHAPTER 66

Guide us, o priests.

--prayer of the student-priest initiates to the God of Internal Medicine

Each week a student-priest presented a case before the chairperson of the Department of Medicine. The meetings were called Ground Rounds, after their host, Lovela Ground. The meetings and the chairwoman were universally feared and dreaded.

The student-priests were deeply divided as to the best time to present a case to the high priest. One school felt that fortune would shine favorably on those who presented early in the quarter. They reasoned that the lack of preparation time as well as relative inexperience in formal presentations would wring mercy from the heart of Lovela Ground. The second school of thought, to which I subscribed, believed that mercy from Ground was capricious at best and probably correlated better with the proximity to lunch than the week of the quarter.

The student-priests assembled quietly, nervously. We took seats around a large round table after the High Priest sat. There were also theories about where to sit during Ground Rounds. As if by silent agreement, we began sitting as far as possible from the chairwoman. One of the few remaining seats was opposite Dr. Ground. Enrique Abraham, the first presenter, took that seat resignedly. Enrique shuffled a small, neat pile of papers. He fingered a perennial patch of pale crimson at the angle of his right jaw. Often when the priest-cadet was subjected to stress, the small reddened island would engulf his entire face. The last seat next to the high priest was filled. The chairwoman spoke.

"Let's see. Since you are all here, I guess we can start now." Ground leaned her large torso over the edge of the table as she lit a cigarette. She looked down at two small pieces of paper before her. One was the class picture. The other was a list of our names. She looked briefly around the room.

I noticed for the first time the face of a student-priest sitting opposite me. She had been a member of my entering class. Her facial feature, her bearing often made me think of a model. She smiled across the table at me in recognition. I smiled back at her. So it was true, I thought. Jana did have to repeat Medicine. I had thought the rumors were false. Jana had always seemed on top of everything, always knew the answers to all the questions.

However, the truth of the rumor was undeniable. Jana's large brown eyes glowed with a confidence which I knew could not be there. I watched her closely for a time. As she lit a cigarette, the well-laid facade broke for an instant. I looked away not wishing Jana to know that I knew her secret.

□ □ □ □

"You must be Abraham." Ground spoke the student priest's name with a disarming, grandmotherly smile. Had it not been for my basic distrust of the priests of my team who ultimately answered to the high priest, my anxiety would have vanished entirely.

The student-priest had an unusual manifestation of hives. Most of the time his skin was smooth and pink. When he became nervous one could trace the marks of his of his fingers as he scratched. If he were particularly stress one could see an entire arm and the bottom of his face erupted in a red raised rash

"Yes." Enrique smiled at the high priest. The tone of Enrique's voice was often rich, resonant like that of the best Shakespearean actors. He made it that way as he addressed the chairwoman.

"What's your first name, Dr. Abraham?"

"Enrique."

"O.K., Enrique. Present your case."

Abraham began in the formal style of the priests of internal medicine. Slowly, methodically he plowed through a speech which he had practiced for hours. Through the student grapevine, I knew that the case to be presented was that of a patient with S.L.E. (systemic lupus erythematosus), a disease whose manifestations were both protean and evanescent. I, like my classmates, had done some reading on the disease. Skin, lungs, kidneys—virtually every organ system was affected by the lesions of S.L.E. Enrique had done well to follow the first rule of formal presentations—he had chosen a topic outside the specialty of the person to whom he was presenting. However, he had ignored the second rule. He had not chosen a topic succinct enough that he could gather information in front of him easily and master it.

Instead the student priest had chosen a subject as broad as all of medicine.

Ground interrupted the student-priest. He scratched a dully growing violet patch on the side of his face. "And what would you expect the sed rate to be at this point, Enrique?"

He looked at her blankly, glanced at the stack of papers in front of him. "I don't know . . . there wasn't one done." Enrique scratched the side of his neck. She looked around the table with an only slightly menacing smile.

There was a hint of a wink in her eye directed not at Abraham, but at the other student-priests, her audience. "I know that, Enrique. But what I want to know is what you thought it was?"

Enrique's nails raked the skin on his wrist. Vainly, he sought an answer among his notes. After a moment he realized that there was none there. "I'm not certain I understand your question."

Ground was enjoying toying with the priest-cadet. "I'll make it easy for you," she purred. "Was as it low, high. Normal?"

Enrique dug his nails savagely into his chest. The entire right side of his face was a large crimson blotch.

"High?" He answered.

"Of course, it was high, wasn't it?" The student-priest began scratching with both hands. "You can continue now."

Enrique began again, shaken. He continued with a long, history of a patient which a devastating disease. He was interrupted frequently by the high priest.

Abraham's finely polished, meticulous presentation became disjointed.

His entire face, arms and chest became one large angry red patch. The student-priest scratched continually with both hands, digging into his itching skin.

His fellow students felt for the tortured priest-cadet as redness crept over his entire body.

Finally, the question we all knew was coming. “Enrique, what did his urinalysis show?”

Finally, a time for the student-priest to shine. We all knew Enrique knew the answer. I knew the answer. Every student sitting at the table knew the answer. Enrique had told us what the urinalysis showed. Shine Enrique!! Shine!

A dejected student-priest priest, head bowed, spoke into the table. “I don't know.”

Looks of pity, disbelief, passed between the student-priests. Abraham looked at the chairwoman, then at his fellow students. I kept my eyes on the table as the last of the student-priest's courage fell.

Noon and the end of the conference arrived, bringing an end to the suffering of one student-priest. The other students present breathed an uneasy sigh of relief.

Each of us knew--our time was coming.

CHAPTER 67

The word doctor comes from the Latin meaning to teach. We must do more than simply practice medicine. Each of us has an obligation to teach it as well.

--lectures, Academy of the Priests of the God of Life

It was perhaps the third week of my tour on 9-west that I began to really notice the continual, senseless, emotional blood-letting, the undeclared, but bitterly fought warfare waged by the priests of 9-West against us, their student charges. Our constant, unjustified belittling in front of both patients and staff was an unquestioned emotional drain. I wondered what we had done to engender such animosity. As I could think of no grave sin we had committed, I thought it nothing more than the student-priest's rite of passage. What bothered me more than the in-fighting was the lack of any organized teaching by the priests who supervised us. I began to wonder, was it that I was missing something or was something missing?

An answer to these questions, came during a hurried lunch with a student from another Internal Medicine team.

A thin man with straight, almost black hair and a neatly trimmed mustache sat across from me as I chomped on my favored dry hamburger and thousand island dressing.

"How do you like your team?" he asked me.

"They're O.K., I guess." I answered vaguely. Some of the dressing splattered on the table before me.

"I hear you guys don't get much teaching." It was a statement, not a question. I did not reply. An avalanche of questions began to have clear, unsettling answers. I finished lunch in thoughtful silence.

□ □ □ □

At times, when 9-West was filled, our team had patients on other wards. We rounded first on our own ward then went to other floors as needed.

On these forays I sometimes lagged behind to observe the working of other teams. I was struck by the camaraderie between the students and priests of other wards. Work was a shared responsibility which was rewarded by teaching and praise. Questions by house officers had an altogether different intent than that to which I had become accustomed. Questions were asked of the student-priests of 9-West solely to ascertain that we had completed a given task for the convenience of the house staff. The often obvious cruelty with which this was done, left little room for doubt of the malicious intent. Almost nothing was explained voluntarily. Our questions were answered either perfunctorily, in clipped mono-syllables, or not at all. All questions were regarded by our house staff as an admission of unexcused ignorance, and as corroboration of our prejudged abject stupidity.

However, on other teams, the questions asked by house staff, were of an illustrative nature. On 9-west we would be asked if we had checked the SGPT, what was its value, nothing more. On other teams, students were asked if one expected the SGPT to change and why? If the correct answer was given, the theme was expanded upon. If an answer was incorrect, the correct answer was explained at length, sometimes with a suggestion of further references. There was no loss of face. My journeys into other wards became longer and more frequent as I became aware of the immense differences between ours and other medicine teams. At first, during these hallway exchanges, I openly listened. However, almost invariably once it was noticed that I was paying attention, the conversation would abruptly end or move to another location. For a time, I thought it only coincidence, but the pattern became altogether too consistent and predictable. I started pretending to read a chart as the conversations took place. I wondered did the jaundiced eye of the priests of internal medicine extended beyond the halls of 9-West.

□ □ □ □

Sometimes when the loneliness, the isolation, the grating of the constant antagonisms overwhelmed me, I succumbed to self-pity. *Why me?* I believed in the priesthood, its healing, its lofty mission. My intentions, my goals were among the most noble known to humankind. I did my work. More, I worked damned hard. I was often on the wards hours after the interns and residents had gone. I knew my patients. I tried.

Why then were the priests so hostile toward me? Why then did they pile petty insult upon petty insult upon gross injustice? When these moods overcame me, the knowledge that I was not alone in my suffering, nor the one singled out for the greatest amount of abuse, gave little solace. When it seemed that I could not face another day with the priests of the God of Internal Medicine, I would call up pages of history, ancient yet new as the gray dawn. I would remember a boy born into slavery, not knowing his father, held in ignorance by the jaws of unjust laws, a boy who bribed and outwitted his young masters to learn first a single letter, a word, a sentence, a book, an entire written language.

I remembered a boy whose command of language earned him a reputation as an inspired editor and one of the finest orators of all time. I remembered a boy who grew to be a man who was consulted by heads of state, a man who was one of the greatest thinkers America has ever produced. I would think of this boy of ignoble beginnings who overcame hardships far greater than any I had ever known. I would think of this boy and find the courage to endure beyond even the priests of 9-West.

CHAPTER 68

The priesthood is the officer corps of the healing arts.
--academy lectures

Samuel Boford's name rolled uncomfortably over the tongue like a lumbering, sluggish vessel setting out on a stormy sea. The name was too close to that of a chain of popular restaurants. The tongue kept confusing the two, enunciating neither clearly, once the other entered one's thoughts. Larry, Mike and I looked around the small conference room. I thought that the room was the wrong one or that the meeting had been canceled. We turned to go.

"Come on in," the room's sole occupant beckoned to us. I looked at my watch. It was seven minutes past the scheduled beginning of the meeting.

"We're here for teaching rounds." Louis spoke.

"You're in the right place." Boford, the student-priest trainer, answered.

Reggie waved a handful of brown hair out of his eyes. "Where's everybody else?" he asked the priest.

"You're it." Boford's voice was edged with anger. We seated ourselves as far from the corpulent priest as politeness and the room's small dimensions would allow. Louis explained that Tim would be present soon. Louis' voice was appeasing. He was always the statesman.

"What?" Boford called.

"Tim, the other student on our team will be here in a few minutes. He's doing a procedure." Louis answered. Schnauzer had insisted that Tim help with the procedure on his patient.

"Humph." Boford's mood was not softened.

I was seated directly in front of the priest. Louis and Reggie sat on either side of me. "Guess we better begin, " the priest said gruffly. The topic was cardiology.

The heart and cardiology held a special interest for me. I was intrigued by the subtle complexities of an organ which was comprised almost exclusively of muscle fibers. The study of the circulatory system had been both the most trying and most exciting portion of the physiology course.

To further my knowledge in this area, I had taken an elective in cardiology with one of the giants of the field. The end result was that cardiology was one of my strong points.

Boford first reviewed the basic physiology. The disease states of the heart followed. As I listened, I recalled old lessons. These I integrated with the new information which the priest gave. As the lecture continued, I realized that something was not quite right. There was a strangeness to the interaction with the priest which took me some time to pin-point. I found the source of my discomfort. During forty minutes of lecturing, the priest had looked only at Reggie. He had not once looked at Louis or me.

After a time, Boford began to use the Socratic method. He asked questions to illuminate a point.

The priest fired a question. I answered. Another question. I answered. He looked only at Rand. He fired a third question. I answered again. The priest did not acknowledge my answer. Look at me, you bastard, I thought, as I answered a fourth and a fifth question. We continued in this vain, with only an occasional question being answered by another student-priest. We continued until the appointed hour of closing when the corpulent priest, filled with himself and an over-abundance of flesh, left.

THE THIRD YEAR

The rage within me was as impenetrable as the walls of the House of the God of Life, as impenetrable as the priest's arrogance and pride. The anger smoldered as I returned to the halls of 9-West and the priests of the God of Internal Medicine.

CHAPTER 69

The use of chemotherapy in the fight against cancer is a case of selective poisoning. One gives treatment with the hope that only diseased tissue will succumb, but, invariably, vitally-needed, normal tissue is destroyed as well.

--Oncology Manual, Battle tactics against cancer

A**s soon as we** were certain, I had asked to tell her. The priests had gladly allowed me the unpleasant task. I did not trust the priests. Too often, I had seen despair, hopelessness, and pain written across the faces of our charges when they had learned, only by accident as we priests intellectualized at their bedside about their condition, that they would soon succumb to the priest-enemy, Death. Too often, I had felt ashamed to be one of the team of doctors caring for a patient who tried desperately to deny or pretend they had not heard what had been said. I had faced the anger and sullenness of patients who knew, though never told, that their death was near. I had, too often, seen the look of betrayal on their faces as they were neglected by nurses and seen for progressively shorter and less frequent visits by house staff. I had volunteered to tell her. I did not trust my fellow priests.

□ □ □ □

"Mrs. Kirkpatrick, how much did Dr. Brown tell you?" Brown was the oncologist following the case. He had seen the patient the previous day.

He said he thought that the x-rays showed some kind of blockage." Her Irish brogue, pleasant and mild, lent an almost playful air to her speech.

"Is that all?" I searched her face for the answer to the question beyond my spoken question. She searched mine for the second question and the statement beyond it.

"Is there more, doctor?" The time was at hand. I could give her no more time. I swallowed heavily. I could not draw out the telling. A searching dread was already full upon her face.

"You have a tumor." I paused. She watched me intently, saying nothing. Her chest rose and fell, deeply, rhythmically. "It's blocking your intestine", I said. "We cannot cure the tumor, but we can relieve the obstruction before it gets worse." I paused, again, giving her time to absorb what I had said. A cart passed the solid wooden door to her room noisily.

"It's cancer, isn't it?"

"Yes." I said as gently as I could.

She sobbed spasmodically as she whispered, "Oh, my God!" Minutes passed.

The hospital's ever constant heart rhythm, intermittent foot falls, some near, some far, some fading, was punctuated by the drone of distant conversation and the random overhead page.

"Forgive me for crying like this. I just can't help it." She spoke between sniffle.

"A good cry will do you good. It's not easy to stand up to what you've stood up to. You've had some very bad news."

□ □ □ □

Days pass. The metastatic work-up continues. Widespread disease is found. Days, nights, on-calls, work rounds, x-ray rounds, patient visits meld.

Mrs. Kirkpatrick says hello. She smiles bravely through pain which holds her in a steel grip. I see not her, but the skeleton of her etched hard and white against the softer gray shadows of her flesh. I see irregular, punched out spots in the lower end of her spine. She tells me that the medicine only takes the edge off her pain. She holds her back as if she sees the image of her in my eyes. The real-life image of this woman appears before me. "*We'll see* if we can give you something stronger", I say, knowing that already her pain is beyond the power of the Gods of Medicine and will grow stronger yet. She cuts on a lamp. I am blinded by the florescent light shining mercilessly through bone which looks like worm-ridden *pieces* of wood. Another hole appears on the x-ray. The woman doubles over with pain. Two wells, her eyes, overflow. She reaches out. Doctor, she says, help me. I am overwhelmed by helplessness. I am not a doctor, yet, I say to myself. My answer seems weak to the immediacy of the moment. Her pain, her torment strikes a chord that cuts through the deception of title, rank, training. She has reached out at a basic level. As I put my arms around her to comfort her, I feel both angry and frightened at the same time. Why did they not teach me how the doctor puts aside the priesthood and becomes the most delicate and humble of creature--a human being?

The woman sobs frantically. I look toward the door, hopefully. Maybe someone will come in as they have so often in the past and tell me what an incompetent fool I am. Perhaps they will show me the right way to comfort this woman. She cries unashamedly, as a child cries. My chest is wet with her tears. The door way looms empty. I realize that truly it does not matter for my teachers would be at a greater loss than I. I feel cheated by those whose learning I respect. I feel lost. I feel like crying uninhibited, as this woman cries. I feel like crying, but no one would understand--not this woman, not the house officers, not my fellow students. No one will understand, but my tears come anyway. The stethoscope slips from my neck, falls to the floor. I feel relieved of an awesome weight.

CHAPTER 70

The social history is an integral part of the evaluation of any patient. It contains a good deal more than where one works and how many children one has.

--a priest of the Joined Hands

Joyce did not want to go home. Our usually agreeable charge had had a tantrum when told that her hospital stay was nearing its end. She had become sullen and depressed, refusing to cooperate with treatment regimens or to take medications. Joyce's acts, so uncharacteristic of her previous behavior, opened a flood gate of emotion among the nurses and aides. Incidents buried by time, but not forgotten, were again related. Many expressed the opinion that our charge deliberately did not take her medications at home so that she would have to be re-admitted. My own patience with Joyce was growing short as well.

While Tim was away caring for his very seriously ill mother, Joyce had been assigned to me. Several times, I had been paged out of a meeting, during the middle of a procedure, or as I was leaving for the day to coax Joyce into cooperating with a test or taking her medication. As the nurses stormed our rounds, Donald, the attending priest, was thrown into the middle of the fray. His shock of straight, black hair and point of a nose turned spasmodically from one speaker to the next. The priest turned to me.

"What do you know about what's going on in her life, right now?" "Well," I shrugged my shoulders, "not much." No one else was able to offer much information, either. As she was for the time my patient, I was assigned the task of finding out what was wrong with our charge. I resented the task, though I knew it was necessary, though I knew that I was the logical choice.

"What do you do for fun?" I asked Joyce. It seemed a logical place to start. I rested my clipboard in my lap, as I leaned back in the plastic-coated chair. Joyce sat erect, but not uncomfortably, in bed.

We-e-ell . . . " Joyce's eyes searched the ceiling. " . . . I just sit around the house mostly."

"Surely, you must do something besides sit around the house." "That's what I do most of the time. Sit around the house and take my medication."

"Don't you have friends you visit or do things with?"

"No." She answered without hesitation.

"Don't you have any hobbies or things you like to do?"

"Like what?" She looked into my face questioningly.

"I don't know . . . Play chess or checkers or jog or something."

"No." The edge of rain clouds gathered about her face.

I tried a different approach. "Do you ever go out?"

She paused thoughtfully. "Go out?"

"Yeah, like on a date."

Her face brightened slightly. "William takes me out sometimes."

Finally! I thought. "Where do you go?"

"Sometimes we go driving."

"Any place in particular?"

"No."

"Where else do you go when you're not out just driving?"

"Sometimes we go to McDonald's." A smile of unabashed joy filled her face.

"You like McDonald's, don't you?"

"Yes. They have good food."

"Do you do anything else fun?"

"No." She answered. The happiness began to drain from her face. I did not pursue the conversation further. Speech became difficult, pouring from my mouth like thick syrup on a cold morning. An overwhelming sadness came upon me. She was a girl, grown into womanhood, yet the highlight of her life outside the hospital was a trip to McDonald's. The self-pity I had regarding my own personal life fled from me like a ghost, shamed and naked before the day.

CHAPTER 71

That patients fall in love with their physicians is both myth and reality. More often, it is the priesthood, rather than the person, that is the object of these feelings. In our dealings with our charges, we must continually bear in mind that they are doubly vulnerable both because of the malady which brought them to us and because of the high regard in which they hold the priesthood. At all times, our actions must be guided by this knowledge and concern for our charge's best interests.

--Academy lectures on Ethics

She has some bleeding from the vagina, doctor." The somber faced mother of Joyce McNair told me. Her features were set in brown stone as she spoke to me. She was unhappy to greet me with this news. I was unhappy to hear it. Vaginal bleeding? Joyce? I had worked feverishly to get my charge out of the hospital, to stabilize the disease which had no cure. Now she was bleeding. My mind turned over a myriad of possibilities. Each of them was hopelessly grave, hopelessly complex. Each required a substantial prolongation of a hospital stay which daily became more taxing. Her disease, infinitely complex in itself, and the necessity of my presence several times a day for even routine matters, was slowly overwhelming the third-year clinical clerk assigned to her.

My thoughts whirled down endless paths of disease, complicated even beyond the reasoning of the gray-haired priests. A headache, something from which I seldom suffered, began to throb as the articulation of nightmares crept into my consciousness. Vaginal bleeding. Joyce. I did not want to believe my ears. Though it was a reality I did not want to accept, I could not deny it. She had vaginal bleeding. She was my charge. I tried to contain the, frustration and anger inside of me. I tried to think logically. If GYN was consulted, it would be a day before they saw her. They would probably shake their heads and throw the problem back to the medicine people. More important than this, she was our charge. I felt obliged to carry the investigation as far as I was able before a consultant was called. Having witnessed the awkward pelvic exam of more than one internist, I knew that I was the best qualified on the team to perform the exam.

□ □ □ □

Joyce was in stirrups. I looked carefully again. Not only could I not locate the site of bleeding, I could find no trace of blood at any site. Perhaps GYN would have to explain the bleeding, after all.

"Where did you say the bleeding was?" I spoke to Joyce.

Her mother answered. "She said it was on the side."

"Where?" I asked again.

"It was on the side, doctor. I looked there myself and I couldn't see much. Just a little scratch."

I looked again. I saw nothing. "Joyce, can you show me where it was that you were bleeding from?"

She half sat up. She wore that same girlish smile I had come to know so well.

"Here." She indicated a large area.

"Joyce, can you show me with one finger where it was bleeding from?"

"Somewhere over here." She smiled contentedly. She was still vague. "That doesn't help me very much."

"Here, let me show you." Joyce's mother stepped forward, throwing back the sheet impatiently. "She showed me before. Here it is, right here, doctor. See, this right here?"

"You certain that's it?"

"Yes, that's it."

I could not believe what I saw. She had indicated a superficial area about twice the size of a match head. The top layer of skin had been scraped away.

"That's just a little scratch. Is that what you were concerned about?" I looked at Joyce, her mother.

"Yes, that's it." The mother answered.

"That's nothing to worry about at all."

Relief shown on the mother's face. Tense shoulders fell as if released from a taunt cable. "That's all. I just wanted y'all to check it."

"Sure. It's nothing at all." I tried to smile through the tightness that was my face.

"Good." The mother spoke.

"Well, Joyce, looks like you can go home now. Everything is fine." I showed a smile, more genuine, this time.

"Come on, let's go, Joyce." Her mother called.

"Bye, Joyce."

She sat up to watch me as I stood to leave. "Bye." She smiled that little girl smile at me once more.

Though I had not thought of it before that moment, Joyce was a girl whom I would have called pretty under different circumstances.

"You take care of yourself, now." I called to her from the door way.

"Bye." She called again. As I turned, she beamed a smile at me of innocence and womanhood, joy and sadness.

As I left, I was touched somewhere deep within, somewhere beyond the robes of the priest.

CHAPTER 72

In the fight against renal disease and hypertension, we must realize their inter-relatedness. We must remember that one often foreshadows the other and that both may arise from a single given cause.
--lectures, House of the God of Internal Medicine

I **remember him** most for his pride and independence. Willie was a thirty-six year old male with both renal failure and hypertension who was admitted to 9-West because of an infection in his left forearm. As my charge was wheeled onto the ward, his head hung slightly. I asked him several questions. His replies were brief, sullen, and hostile. Though this was my first meeting with my charge, his mood surprised me. Willie was known for his congenial cheerfulness. As an ill-appearing Willie was placed in bed, a steady barrage of visitors, led by a priest of the renal service, began. He was followed by several more priests, nurses, well-wishers. I waited impatiently for them to finish. As dusk approached and the visitors showed no signs of relenting, I decided to complete the examination of my charge in the morning.

□ □ □ □

It was afternoon before I saw Willie again. As he wheeled himself back to his room, shunning aid, I was impressed that he did not appear as sick as he had the previous night. His black. hair was neatly combed. He spoke to me as he passed. I answered non-committedly. As soon as he entered his room, he drew me into a gregarious conversation. We spoke at length.

I soon grew to like Willie. More I respected him. I learned that though my charge had a disease which required that he be linked to a hemodialysis machine for five hours, three times a week, he managed to maintain a full-time job. His insistence on working when he could have easily been placed on disability as most renal patients, was but one of the ways in which Willie manifested an aggressive independence. He was active in all phases of his care. His determined adaptation to a devastating disease which crippled lesser spirits, was remarkable. As anyone who knew Willie soon found, his greatest source of pride, the object of his devout adoration, was his daughter. He showed me her picture. She was an attractive girl with large, free-flowing curls.

"She's eighteen." He smiled. "She's pretty, ain't she?"

"Yes." I agreed. We talked a while longer before another visitor came. I took my leave. I thought it strange the almost total personality change in so short a span of time.

As time passed, I saw this recur several times. It was a while before I found that marked personality changes was common in renal patients. Further, their mood was highest just after dialysis and lowest just before.

I observed my charge closely. Indeed, his moods showed such a variation. I was grateful that a useful secret was unfolded to me.

CHAPTER 73

Suicide, depression, divorce are but a few of the ways in which stress takes its toll on the lives of physicians. Driving the toll yet higher is denial, which often delays or altogether prevents treatment. The presence together of stress and denial causes immeasurable suffering of physicians, their family, friends, co-workers.

For the sake of our loved ones, our patients, our co-workers, ourselves, we need to abandon the image of the physician-priest as super-human and find an effective means of stemming this untreated and unacknowledged scourge.

--the Heretic Priest, Healing priests healing patients

We were fighting--again. Loudly--again. The idyllic first three weeks of our reunion was followed by constant arguments. Grace and I fought over many things, large and small. However, most of the conflict revolved around the relationships each of us had had while we had been apart.

Suspicion, distrust, envy were festering sores made more purulent by our endless bickering. Though I loved with my bride, my lover, my friend, the woman with whom I had spent the happiest moments of my life, I was lonely. I was lonely inside in a way I had not experienced on the longest, pain-ridden day on which I cried for my love. It was a sad and deep loneliness I felt which I could neither run from nor lessen. It gnawed at the edges of my soul as a cancer-like ghoul, unsated and growing.

Loneliness was a never-tiring, patiently voracious beast. hard, unfeeling coldness grew within me. I was dying inside.

On one of the few days in which we did not fight, I heard a knocking at the door. A woman whose face always reminded me of that of the grandmotherly matron in a famous American painting stood outside the screen door. She was my next-door neighbor and one of the owners of the complex. From a frame of silver gray hair she told me that my apartment was needed for an ailing relative. Would I please leave at the end of the month she asked, politely, genteelly? We both knew she lied. However, I was not fighting that day, not with Grace, not with the grandmotherly woman. I could not see the woman's face, only the silver-gray hair and the hole where her smile was. I thanked her, equally politely, and closed the door.

My stomach tightened for only a second, then relaxed. The coldness took another bite. I could feel it growing bigger.

CHAPTER 74

In order to unlock the secret of the auto-immune disorders, we must unlock the secret of the immune system itself.

--lectures, House of the God of Internal Medicine

There was a commotion in the hallway. A half dozen voices could be heard. I was busy but pushed my head through the door to see what was going on. "Stand back, please!" Schnauzer spoke to several people who stood in the hallway.

"Please, move out of the way. We have a sick patient here," another member of the procession called out. Six people in total, including Schnauzer, accompanied a pale, sallow skinned young woman. She appeared pained and grimaced silently. The group turned into a room near the end of the corridor. The last of the entourage was a white-coated figure who held aloft an I.V. bottle as the flame of the

statue of liberty as he disappeared into the bustle of activity. Hanging at the edge of the door (student-priests were not allowed in the room), I learned that the latest charge of the 9-West team had scleroderma and had become hypotensive after a percutaneous renal biopsy. The chart was sequestered at the nurse's station. I had more than enough work to keep me busy. As I turned away from the forbidden doorway to continue my daily ward chores, I became aware of one more fact. I was up for the next admission. That meant that the hypotensive woman with scleroderma was mine.

The morning sun cast a yellow tint into the room. My charge lay with her eyes closed, trying unsuccessfully to sleep. Soon she would be bombarded with medications. Already, the cart containing the slew of pills she was taking, approached.

"Hello." I told the woman my name. "I'll be part of the team of doctors taking care of you." • She opened her eyes, regarding me with the same sour expression that I had seen the day before as she had been wheeled onto 9-West. In the silent instant our eyes met, however, I was able to read a much deeper level of animosity.

"Go away. Don't bother me, . . ." She stopped short of saying the word which had been in her mind. I saw a hate-filled expression, one which I had seen so many times before in the face of bared racial prejudice. I had never experienced this from a patient.

Had it been earlier in the third year, I would probably have turned and gone away. However, I knew my worth, particularly to a patient like her. I would be called to draw blood and handle any other problem the nurses could not take care of, not the intern, not the resident. I was also angered that as sick as she was, as much as she needed the help of all of the priests of 9-West, she could allow something as silly as bigotry to stand in the way of her care. Already, I held a lab slip in my hand for blood that the blood drawers could not draw. It was a blood count. She was bleeding and needed the test desperately if she were not to bleed to death.

"I don't understand English." She called to me, waving me away disgustedly.

"Yo hablo Español." (I speak Spanish, I said with an almost perfect accent.) My Spanish was not that good. I played a bluff with a perfect poker face.

"I don't want no more tests." She spoke in clear English.

I put the tourniquet on her arm. I did not ask permission. "The fact of the matter is that you are bleeding quite rapidly." I looked deep into her face. She turned away. I continued searching for a vein.

"If we do not have this blood test, we will not know how much blood to give you and you may bleed to death." I spoke as sternly as I could.

"Alright, alright, just take the blood test."

As I searched her arms, I glanced at my watch. Attending rounds, at which my presence was required, would be starting soon. She had no obvious veins. She sighed impatiently, as I searched the other arm. I ignored her.

"You're going to feel a stick now." I removed the cover from the syringe.

"They already stuck me there this morning. They couldn't get nothing." Her face formed a twisted frown. A sigh escaped my lips as I put the syringe back in my pocket. I searched a few minutes more. Nothing. I found nothing else except the site my charge did not want one to try. Usually, I listened to patients when they told me such things. They were usually right.

"I'm sorry," I explained to my charge, "I have to go where I can at least feel a vein. This is the only place on you unless I go to your groin. And I don't want to do that, if at all possible."

"Nobody's going to take no blood from me down there!" She spoke loudly, emphatically.

"Well, then?" I shrugged. She sucked her tongue, disgustedly.

I tightened the tourniquet. A tense moment passed.

To the surprise of both Rosario Guerra and her assigned student-priest, blood flowed freely into the syringe with my first attempt. I said nothing, but smiled inwardly. There was begrudging respect in my patient's eyes.

I left for rounds quickly.

CHAPTER 75

Priest, heal yourself.
--a priest of the Joined Hands

I had decided. I sat in a well-manicures patch of grass outside my apartment, absorbing the cool mid-winter sunshine. There were too many well-founded doubts, too many reasons that we were no longer right together. The good things seemed to have vanished. Tension hung over me. The high level of it in my life was destroying me. There were too many battles, too many obstacles to overcome. Singly, I could win against any. Together they were too much. I was disorganized, hastily retreating, losing, losing pieces of me. Fighting the priests of the God of Internal Medicine for more than eighty hours a week, fighting with my wife until bedtime, looking for, renting another apartment, and remaining sane were more than I could handle.

However, I knew something that the priests of Internal Medicine, Grace, my grandmotherly land lady did not know. Pressure brought out the best and the worst in me. Once I was in full battle mode, I would win. At times such as these, I hated the person I became. Hard times required hard decisions. Hard times also brought out the hardness in me. I became the Stone Man.

My thought processes went into a coldly logical, largely unfeeling, mechanical mode. Priorities were set, goals clearly delineated. When all was said and done, I could live on the streets if needed, or survive the final dissolution of a marriage which I felt in my gut was beyond reconciliation, but I wanted with all my heart to be a priest.

Decisions, came easily, matter-of-fact-ly.

The priests of 9-West were going to receive what they gave. I would make certain that I had every lab value, the answer to every question I could anticipate. If, per chance, I did not have the answer, they would never catch me with the same question again. I would answer the intern, resident, attending priest snide remark for snide remark. Silly giggles and askance glances would slide like water over my glistening and newly oiled steel skin. I would no longer work through conferences to perform chores that were rightfully theirs. I would learn despite the priests of 9-West. I would learn well.

Next the apartment. It was the least important in the series of crises engulfing me. I could well delay dealing with it until after Medicine 1.

What of Grace and I and our troubled marriage? I viewed it calmly, almost through the eyes of a stranger. The hurts were deep on both sides as was the love. However, while the love waned, the hurt stayed the same. It seemed that each of us had formed an unwholesome dependence upon the other. It was not the dependence born of the love between a man and a woman. Such would been beautiful, healthy, something upon which to build stronger, deeper. Our dependence was based upon the weaknesses of each. Greatest among these was our fear of loneliness. Though honesty hurt, avoiding it was more painful. I loved my ebony-skinned bride. I did not want to be married to her. It was decided.

The responsibility and the consequences, good or bad, were totally mine. Grace, and I would be no more. There was a tightness in my muscles as I waited for the flood of pain and fear that I was sure would immediately overcome me. After a moment, I relaxed. As I sat in the warming winter sun, I was surprised to feel relief. A calm and detached sadness settled over me for I knew that I had made the right decision.

THE THIRD YEAR

CHAPTER 76

The practice of medicine is very much a system of bartering or gambling. The inconvenience, cost, and side effects of a given medication are weighed against the alleviation it affords. The pain and ill-effects of surgery are weighed against the risks of leaving the diseased organ intact. The priest is often nothing more than a seasoned gambler, knowledgeable about risks.

--a priest of the God of Internal Medicine

She was frightened, I knew. Her fear, however, was clothed in an armor of impenetrable hostility. The only way I could communicate with her was by seeming colder and harder than she. She seemed to respect this facade, or, at least, she allowed me to do what I had to do. The pretense took a great deal out of me. It was beginning to wear me down. I listened with annoyance as the intern spoke of the escalation of Guerra's non-compliance with her treatment regimen. She was at veritable war with the nursing and house staff. My jaws tightened as the attending priest cast a glance my way, preparatory to asking me, as he had so many times in the past, to obtain Guerra's consent for another test. The intern continued speaking of his difficulties with our charge.

" . . . She wants to have a baby." I had lost the first part of the sentence in my angry ruminations.

"She wants to have a baby?" I asked.

"Yeah, she does."

"Hm-m-m." I said nothing more. Though I knew that she had had a miscarriage two years previously, I did not know that she still desired a child. This had never come out in any of our talks where I had tried to establish a more cordial relationship with our charge.

A new set of possibilities turned over in my mind.

"Hello." I spoke to my charge, whose unwrinkled, leather-like skin gave her at once the look of unblossomed youth and enduring age. Her disease, sometimes called scleroderma, made even the lines evoked by a smile difficult to discern. This effect of the disease only accentuated her sour expression. She regarded me carefully through mistrustful brown eyes. She looked quickly to my hands, then to the pockets of my white coat for blood drawing equipment. I had none.

"Hello." As she spoke. She relaxed a bit. I could see depression beyond the outer shell of hostility. I had seen this before, but there was a deeper sadness perceptible even through her lineless face. As so often before, my anger at may hostile charge melted when I saw the utter vulnerability and sadness in her eyes. I pulled up a chair.

Often, I played a game with her. I would burst into the room with obvious impatience and self-importance, glance at my watch several times, mutter something about the work I had yet to do, rush through the exam or the taking of a blood sample and leave. I wondered was it in these daily invasions or the less frequent times, usually in the afternoon, when I would sit down, make small talk, try to find out what was on her mind, that allowed me to form the minimal rapport which the other members of the team were unable to form with her. She was lonely. Sometimes it was painfully obvious. Outside of her husband, she had few visitors. Her few close friends and family seldom visited.

"You don't seem your usual self today." I ventured. She said nothing, just looked away from me out the window then into her lap. Water welled within her eyes, but did not fall.

"What's the matter? What's bothering you?"

She spoke to the bed. "I don't want to be in the hospital no more." She regained some composure, raised her head. "I'm tired of being here, tired of all the tests, tired of all the doctors, tired of everything!"

I was set to give her a long lecture about the necessity of her hospitalization and tests, about how the nurses, doctors, everyone were working for her good, about how truly ill she was. However, a moment's reflection upon the series of disasters which had made her hospital course one protracted crisis made me realize that she was right—it was time for her to go home.

We spoke quietly for a time. It was one of few times that there was actually an exchange between us. We spoke of her wanting to have a baby. There was a tenderness in her I had never seen. I told her the truth, that with her current lack of medical control, she could never expect to carry pregnancy to term. If she wanted a baby, all of us, she, her doctors, nurses would have to work together. Tiredness clung to her husky voice. The price she extracted for her consent to this last procedure was my promise to push for her to go home as soon as possible and complete her evaluation as an out-patient.

We ended the conversation with each of us having found new respect and regard for the other. At attending rounds two days later, Mrs. Guerra was again the topic of discussion. Before I spoke, the priests of 9-West had decided that it was time for my charge to leave the House of the God of Internal Medicine. Their reasons were different from Mrs. Guerra's, from mine, but it did not matter. My promise to my charge had been fulfilled. I smiled with an ease with which she could not smile, both for her and for me.

CHAPTER 77

Though they can be found anywhere, infections in the elderly are usually limited to a very few organ systems.

--a priest of the God of Internal Medicine

W**here's that** good-looking colored boy?" She asked as I examined her. She spoke of Tim. Though I rankled at her referring to my colleague as "colored boy", I could not help but smile, amused.

"He had an illness in the family." I explained. "He'll be gone for a little while."

She looked at me with eyes, altogether too bright for her sixty-eight years. "Well, I hope everything goes O.K. with him." She, as all of Tim's patients, had become attached to him.

"Un-huh.". I hummed as I placed the stethoscope on her chest. Bonita Aaron was being treated for a urinary tract infection. She was a vivacious lady who loved the service of hospitals. She had no home, no family. Her pleasant chatter was shared with anyone who was willing to listen and a few who were not. What should have been a ten minute visit had lasted thirty minutes before I knew the time had passed. The meeting ended abruptly when I was summoned by an irate intern who was asking after my assigned tasks.

"Mrs. Aaron, I really have to go now." I said I edged toward the door.

"Wait a minute," she chided good-naturedly, "I haven't finished talking to you."

"Mrs. Aaron, I really do have to go."

"You just got here!" Indeed, it felt that way. "Sorry, Mrs. Aaron. See you later."

"What do you mean, she hasn't voided it two days?" I spoke to Carol, a 9-West nurse.

"She says she hasn't voided since the day before yesterday. Then again, she hasn't taken in that much either."

"Shoot!"

I went to Bonita Aaron's room. She brightened at my approach.

"Mrs. Aaron?"

"Yes, dear." Something about the way she said "dear" made it seem as if she spoke to one of her grand-children, rather than one of the team of doctors taking care of her.

"What's this I hear about you not urinating?"

"Oh, yes," she spoke matter-of-factly, "I haven't gone since Tuesday." (It was Thursday as we spoke.)

In the cramped four-bed room, there was no chair, nor space to put it if I had found one. I sat on the bed beside Bonita Aaron. Her problem necessitated a litany of questions. Mrs. Aaron answered excitedly, with no small amount of excess verbiage. She placed her hand on my knee. As we spoke, it kept creeping up the inner aspect of my thigh. Though I was certain that she meant nothing by it, her hand made me uncomfortable. Very casually, I grasped her in mine, held it for a moment, then deposited it gently into her lap.

The questions continued. The hand, magically reappeared on my leg and again began its forward migration. Again, I grasped it. As I was placing it back in her lap, obliquely and I thought without her knowledge, her voice reached a razor pitch.

"And you leave my hand alone!" She scolded earnestly. "I can put my hand wherever I want it!"

I laughed heartily. Though piqued, she laughed with me. I attempted to renew my questions, but could not. My laughter would not let me begin a single word. For several minutes our laughter was the only sound to be heard. As I exited the room, Carol was writing at the nurse's station.

"You want her cathed?" she asked.

"Yes."

"O.K., write the order and I'll do it." I was surprised that she had not forced me to get the intern to co-sign the order before carrying it out.

"What's so funny?" Carol asked me.

"Nothing, nothing."

□ □ □ □

A few minutes later, I passed the room of Bonita Aaron.

My patient lay, hands behind her head, not smiling, but beaming. Her wiry legs were spread wide apart as Carol put the plastic tube into her bladder.

Seeing her in that position made my laughter begin again. It did not stop even as I reached home that night. A snicker cascaded into a roar of laughter within me.

CHAPTER 78

When to admit? When to discharge? There are few hard indications for either. Most often the decision lies in the gray zone of judgment.

--lectures, House of the God
of Internal Medicine

Bonita Aaron, the loquacious, peppery, sixty-eight year old, was crying. Her tears, like her continual conversation, were unabashed, unpretentious. For two weeks she had been quite well, cured of her urinary tract infection. She had been waiting on a bed in a nursing home. One had been found. In a week it would be ready. Bonita Aaron's eyes were red as well as brown.

"I'm sure you'll like it there, Mrs. Aaron." I told her.

"I won't go! I won't go!" She spoke in the tone of a child throwing a temper tantrum.

"I'm sure it's a nice place."

"I'm going to stay right here." She grabbed the bed railing for emphasis, locking her arm within its frame.

"But Mrs. Aaron, you have to go."

"I'll cry." Her tears began a fresh down pour.

"Oh, *Mrs. Aaron!*" I finally shouted in a final fit of exasperation. The stream of tears continued.

"Well, you don't have to go today, anyway." I tried to placate her.

"I don't have to go?" She looked up at me hopefully.

"Not today. You can stay a little while." How little a while, I did not say. I hoped she would not ask.

"Well," she looked up at me with still reddened brown eyes, but beaming her usual impish smile, "then may I have lunch now?" After talking, her next favorite pastime was eating.

"The lunch trays won't be up for another half-hour." Then as an afterthought, I added, "You know that better than I do."

"Oh, yeah."

"Well, I've got to go, now."

"O.K." She was all smiles again. Other than her reddened eyes, there was no hint that she had been crying just moments before. My mind was drawn back to a single unsubstantiated note in her old chart indicating that my charge had a psychiatric disorder. Was it true, perhaps? I did not know. I had more important things about which to worry.

• * * * *

Her mood as well as mine was sullen. Someone had gotten the inspiration that I should accompany Mrs. Aaron to the nursing home. I felt no small amount of resentment at having been given again the dirty work of the priests of 9-West. Beside me, in the back seat of the cab, sat Linda Aaron.

"Hey, doc, you know where this place is?" The driver spoke to me.

"No. I don't."

"I been there before, but that was a while ago." He bent over a map for a moment. "O.K., here we go."

He eased the car forward. I looked over at my usually talkative charge. She was silent. Tears clouded her eyes. She wore a sad, pity-evoking expression. We passed along Canon's expressways for an indeterminate span of time. The car stopped.

"I think this is it, doc." The sign in front of the building was ambiguous.

"Wait here a moment while I check." I exited the cab.

Inside seemed dark compared to the brightness of the day. My eyes adjusted after a moment. A woman in her mid-fifties sat behind a high counter. I looked around me as I walked toward her. The place was clean, at least. I could not see any of the patient rooms.

"May I help you?" the woman asked.

"Yes. Is this the nursing home?"

"Yes, it is. Are you here to see a patient?"

"No, I've brought a patient. I believe you're expecting her. Bonita Aaron."

"Oh yes. We're expecting her."

"She's outside. I'll go get her."

"O.K." She picked up the phone.

Bonita Aaron walked into the building with only the smallest bit of reluctance. She stopped as she reached the counter. I followed with two small bags that contained all of her belongings.

A very pleasant woman, wearing a white uniform and an air of authority, came from behind a door. Bonita Aaron and I turned to look. The woman spoke to me. "I'll take those from you." I handed her the pieces of luggage. "Hello, Linda. I'm Joanne Worth."

"Hi." It was the first time I had heard her speak all day. She managed a hint of a smile for a second, then returned to her sad expression.

"If you'll come with me, I'll show you your room." The woman turned. Bonita Aaron followed. For a moment, I considered going with her to see her as far as her new room. I thought better of the idea. I would only be prolonging the agony.

"Goodbye, Mrs. Aaron." I called.

"Bye." she called back. I could see the side of her face as a single tear made its way slowly to her chin. The door closed heavily behind her. Feelings of helplessness and guilt gnawed at my insides as the cab moved slowly back to the University Hospital.

CHAPTER 79

Guide us swiftly, surely.
Let not pride nor fear cloud our judgment.
--prayer to the God of Internal Medicine

The big stoic man, with the disease which no one could figure out, was sick. He said nothing, only stared at the ceiling and looked ill. He was Reggie's patient, but all the student-priests, nurses, the aides worried that Apollo was sick and getting worse. Apollo was afflicted by systemic lupus erythematosis, called simply lupus by those in the House of Life. He was an enigma. He was over six-feet tall, two-hundred pounds—and healthy appearing. At least he was until one looked into his dark brown eyes clouded with suffering and pain, until one happened into his room as he moaned when he thought no one was there. His belly hurt him, but why?

"They should call a surgical consult." Reggie protested. Internists were as reluctant to turn their patients over to the surgeons as the priests of surgery were willing to give theirs over to the internists. There was always a feeling of failure, inadequacy when the priests of the God of Internal Medicine transferred a patient.

Reggie stood at the door of Apollo's room. He held a lab slip which had been left because the blood drawers had been unable to draw the sample. Reggie shook the lab slip as he spoke to Tim, Louis, and me.

"He's sick, man." He almost shouted in exasperation. We looked at the large man lying on the bed and agreed in silence. His belly was getting worse. "Want to give me a hand drawing some blood?" Reggie stepped into the room.

"Sure." Tim answered, his voice gentle. Both Tim and Louis followed Reggie into the room. I moved down the hall, deciding to work elsewhere as I was not needed.

A few minutes later, the three student-priests exited the room, spirits and eyes downcast. Reggie spoke to me. "You want to see if you can get some blood?"

"We tried and we couldn't get nothing." Louis added. The interns and resident were off the floor. Besides, we had come to rely almost totally on ourselves. It was surprising how well we managed.

"Sure." I left my clip board at the nurse's station. Several minutes passed as I placed the tourniquet on first one arm, then the other.

"Un poquito dolor." A little pain, I told him in Spanish. Apollo nodded.

The syringe remained empty. A fourth student-priest left the big man's room, dejected.

□ □ □ □

Four student-priests were in the conference room-storage room-lounge. "They should call a surgical consult. He needs an operation." Reggie paced angrily as he spoke.

"Did you talk to Schnauzer about it?" I asked.

"Snot-face?!" Mike turned. "He says not yet. What's he waiting for, for the guy to crump?" Reggie made an obscene waving, pushing gesture, dismissing the resident-priest. "I feel like squashing his friggin' head against the wall. Just get him in a dark alley and beat the living crap out of him." Rand made punching moves against the wall as if he actually had the resident cornered and cowering before him.

We laughed heartily.

□ □ □ □

The next morning, as I darted in and out of rooms, I saw one of the surgical teams approaching. The resident I knew. He had been an international track star and a proctor in the medical school's physiology course. I exchanged warm greetings with him, then returned quickly to my work.

Within a few hours, Apollo was in the operating room. I learned later that Reggie Rand had performed what, for a third year clerk, was a singular act of courage. He had called a consult against the express orders of his resident.

For Apollo, however, it was too late. The strong man, the stoic man, the man with suffering as deep as his brown eyes, was dead within a week.

CHAPTER 80

Pray for good fortune.
--a priest of the God of Life

Painless jaundice. These two words together denoted hopelessly grave possibilities. Eros Farmer, a thirty-eight year old man who spoke with a soft mid-western accent made even softer by years of living in Northeastern and West coast cities, Eros Farmer, who had injected heroine and anything else he could get his hands on into veins hardened like adobe brick, Eros Farmer, veteran of a thousand hustles, liver of the good life, the low life, consummate story teller, yarn spinner, survivor of a hundred infections and imprisonments which had killed all his friends his own age who had lived as he, this man about whom volumes could be written, was summed up in two small words, sixteen letters--painless jaundice.

Daily, as the evidence mounted, the priests of 9-West passed Mr. Farmer's bed. He cast distant side-wise glances at the priests as if seeing them and not seeing them at the same time. They in turn, regarded him just as distantly. To them, he was an interesting case, but first and always a junkie, a vulpine seeker of pain medication, one of legions of manipulative and knowledgeable falsifiers of illness who would stop at nothing to get another injection of narcotics, another fix. The priests of 9-West were aloof, distant, distrustful. It was clear that the distrust was mutual. I, myself, did not fully trust Eros Farmer, but I liked him. He spoke to me quite honestly most of the time. As the ritual work rounds passed his bed daily, he would watch the priests silently, through large jaundiced eyes. Then as they passed, I smiled or touched or winked at him. He would smile back at me. He asked me few questions. I was glad. From the onset, it did not look good for him. With the results of each test, the outlook got worse. We discussed a myriad of diagnostic procedures for Mr. Farmer. Finally, we decided that the best for our charge was the ultrasound. It was then new. Canon was one of the premier centers for this new form of imaging. Each day as we waited for Eros Farmer's turn on the crowded schedule, another benign cause of our charge's deeply jaundiced eyes was ruled out. The house staff continued to discuss this "very interesting case", as often as not, within hearing of the patient. I watched with discomfort as apprehension, then controlled terror showed on the face of my charge.

The ultrasound was performed. The worse was confirmed. None of the priests told the patient. As the all-important diagnosis had been made, concern with Eros Farmer, the adroit survivor, the veteran of a score of hospital admissions and twice as many teams of house staff, vanished rapidly.

Annoyance played upon my mind. I was angered that neither the house staff, nor the attending priest had told the patient of his diagnosis, yet I was relieved as well. I had seen them face the priest-enemy, Death, before. They were neither gracious, nor humane in the face of defeat. I asked for, and was gladly granted permission to tell the patient of his diagnosis. Eros Farmer was not the only one who distrusted the priests of 9-West.

The four-bedded room was empty except for the two of us. As many times before, we spoke of small unimportant things.

Somehow, we were speaking of his disease before I had intended.

Louis passed in the hallway. Eros Farmer and I both looked up as his footsteps approached and receded.

"Doc, you know, before I got sick, I used to be as light as that boy there." He pointed to where Louis had just passed. My charge looked at me quite seriously from eyes so deeply jaundiced that they were no longer yellow, but orange. He must have read the look of incredulity on my face as I smiled, for he added quickly, "Really!" On my first meeting with Louis, I had thought he was of strictly European ancestry. Mr. Farmer's skin was of the darkest ebony. No amount of jaundice could have ever caused such a change.

"Really?" I smiled again as I admitted that I could not help but be taken by his childish charm even as he stretched the truth beyond endurance. I thought again, I like him. With all that I know of him, I like him. The curtain made a dragging, rolling sound as I pulled it close. Sitting forward on the edge of my chair, I could think' of no way to delay or soften what I had come to tell him.

"Mr. Farmer, . . . " I paused searching the ceiling for an eloquent, soothing, gentle phrase. I had selected words to say earlier, but as always, when face to face with the patient, pre-selected phrases did not seem appropriate. " . . . Mr. Farmer." Again, words did not flow. He looked at me questioningly, apprehensively. I swore at myself under my breath. "Mr. Farmer," I began again, "we've completed most of the tests, now." He stared at me anxiously through orange eyes. "We're pretty certain what's going on . . ."

"Yeah, doc?"

I suddenly realized that I would have to explain some basic anatomy and physiology before he could understand what I was about to say. "Mr. Farmer, do you know what your pancreas is?"

"Not exactly. I heard of it."

"Let me show you." I pulled out my pen, began drawing on the bed sheet, then thought better of it. He would probably want a record he could keep. I pulled a sheet of paper from my note pad. Slowly, putting in just enough detail for him to understand, I explained where the bile was blocked and why he was jaundiced. I paused, waiting for him to absorb what I had said. His eyes showed me he understood.

"The reason there is a blockage, Mr. Farmer, is that you have a cancer in the pancreas." He looked at my drawing, said nothing for a moment.

"Somehow, I figured that was what I had." His jaundiced eyes looked into mine, searchingly. I knew and was prepared for the next question.

"Can they do anything about it, doc?"

"The cancer you have is a very fast growing one." I told him. "Already it has spread beyond the pancreas. Later on, there are procedures which might make you more comfortable, relieve some of the jaundice and itching, but there is no cure. It's beyond that."

He looked into the blankness of the drawn drape, his expression just as vacant. I eased back in my chair.

A moment passed. "Do you want to ask me any questions?"

"No, doc." I sensed that he wanted to be alone.

"Well, if you have any questions, don't hesitate to call for me." I rose. "Do you want the curtain open?"

"No, it's fine like it is."

"See you."

"O.K., doc."

I looked back at my charge. This survivor of a thousand games and of a life so hard, it had destroyed lesser men, had finally met a misfortune he could not overcome. Watching him was not pleasant. I felt empty, powerless, disgusted. I felt disgust at my own inability to help this man, at the smug callousness of the priests of 9-West, at Death. Too many of my patients were dying.

On my previous two clerkships, only one of my patients had died, a burnt-out alcoholic who presented more dead than alive, bloated almost beyond recognition as even human. I had seen him only once before he was transferred to the ICU and died.

On Medicine, patients died seemingly daily. But they were more than patients, they were *people*. Disgust and anger welled within me. An intern asked me to perform a minor task. I glared at him for no reason. I hurried through my work. Leaving early, I let the doors of the House of the God of Life, the God of Healing close behind me. Perhaps, I could find an affirmation of life in the newly-green blades of grass pushing upward in anticipation of spring.

CHAPTER 81

Medicine cannot be learned from books. It must be taught by those who practice it.
--academy lectures

It was the end of my fifth week, nearly my last week at the U. I came in answer to the summons of Marvin Stand, course director for Medicine 1. The note said that I was to meet Stand in his office at the V.A. Hospital at one-thirty.

The shuttle bus between the V.A. and the U. made only hourly trips during lunch time. I arrived at the V.A. An hour early in order to avoid being a few minutes late. The note was clear--meet Dr. Stand at his office at One-thirty in the afternoon. Beyond the note, however, loomed vague and unpleasant uncertainty. What did he want?

The sun peaked between clouds, intermittently, as the minibus came to a halt in front of the Canon Veterans Administration Hospital. The hospital was called simply, "the V.A.", by the priests of the House of Life. The door slammed behind me. The bus moved on. I drew my white coat, the short white coat of the student-priest and intern, close to me. There was a pervasive chill. My hands, however, were colder than the cloudy, wind-swept day.

As I approached, the automatic doors of the main entrance opened like the jaws of a rapacious beast. I moved within.

There were a few people in. the cafeteria whom I knew. I chose to sit at a table alone. I stirred the ice of my soda, idly. Though my stomach gurgled intermittently, I was neither hungry nor thirsty. I decided to wait the last half-hour before my appointment in the course director's office.

The doors of the elevator closed, leaving me in the common central area of the four-winged hospital complex. I walked several yards to Stand's office.

"May I help you?" a woman with short, neatly cut, dark brown hair looked up from her typing. Her tone was pleasant, business-like.

"Yes." I glanced around the office. I told her my name.

"I'm here to see Dr. Stand."

"Just a minute, I'll page him."

"No, no. That's O.K." I protested. "My appointment is not till one-thirty."

"I'll page him and see if he is free now." She was polite, insistent. "O.K." I said doubtfully.

"Hi." Come on in. Stand waved me into his office as he held the door. He flashed a genuine and unabashed boyish smile.

"Come on in, sit down." He closed the door. The priest appeared surprisingly young despite his totally white hair. Lowering myself into the chair, I felt no less ill at ease. The priest stood behind his desk, looking at a stack of papers as he pulled off his coat.

"Excuse me just one minute." He picked up one of the stacks of papers, carried them to his secretary, then returned.

"Sorry you had to wait. I was just finishing up rounds." I wondered did he realize that I was early. I said nothing. "Let's see, now." He picked up a manila folder. It contained several sheets of paper. He was obviously familiar with what the file contained as he browsed a few seconds to refresh his memory.

"Things not going too well on Medicine, huh?" He looked at me as he spoke. There was another question or a statement beyond his question which I could not read.

"O.K., I guess." I was non-committal. He looked at me earnestly.

"You've seen these already, haven't you?" he indicated the papers within the file. I had been trying, unsuccessfully, to steal a look at them.

"What are they?"

"Your six-week evaluations."

"No, I haven't seen them."

"Oh." His voice demeanor was apologetic. He handed the file to me. "Then, you'd better take a look at them." I took the papers. "I'll give you a few minutes to look over them." My name was typed neatly across the tab of the folder. Inside were three pages of a printed form, followed by a half-page narrative. Stand went in and out of his office a few times, then sat at his desk writing. He glanced up at me a few times. It took me a few minutes to decipher the code.

There were some twenty or so categories which formed the basis of evaluation. These included everything from appearance, to relationship with house staff, patients, knowledge of basic sciences, clinical medicine, to attitude and quality of written work. One could be evaluated as outstanding, above average, average, needs improvement, and unsatisfactory. Though we were in a pass-fail system, the scale bore an amazing resemblance to the A-B-C-D-F system I had known all my life. What I saw before me was a composite of several forms like the one I held. Letters ("A" for attending, "R" for resident, "I" for intern) denoted the rank of the person giving a specific mark. Evaluators were not identified beyond this. I could feel the muscles in my face tighten as I realized the meaning of what had been written. There were perhaps two or three marks in the column labeled above average, several under average. The bulk were, however, under improvement needed. I was further piqued at a few marks in the unsatisfactory column. Anger welled as a flood within me. A thousand expletives raced across my mind, but none reached my lips. I looked once again at the papers before me, this time seeking out the letter "A" for attending. Those marks could only belong to Donald. I was surprised that his marks were the worst. He had evaluated several categories of my write-ups as unsatisfactory. My write-ups had always been rated "very good" or "excellent" by my resident. Donald had never seen one of my write-ups. I turned to the narrative section which consisted of direct quotes from several evaluators. There were no charges of laziness, ignorance, nor any other specific short-comings. Instead, I was labeled an indefinably poor student. My mind boiled. I laid down the paper, trying to contain an outburst only a heartbeat away. I drew in a deep breath and looked into the cool blue eyes of Marvin Stand.

"Some problems there, huh?" The priest spoke calmly.

"Yes." I looked down at the desk, trying to control my anger. Several minutes passed before I could look him in the face again without exploding.

Stand asked how did I feel about my clerkship experience, about my evaluations? I told him honestly how I felt, not because I thought that he actually cared about the difficulties of the student-priests of 9-West, but because it was the only way I could control the anger, the unbridled rage which threatened to engulf me there in his office. I told him of the unreasoned antagonism between the student-priests and the house staff of 9-West. I told him of the total abrogation by the priests of their responsibility to teach. I told him of the duplicity involved in the written feed-back we received and the pages before me. I was surprised that he listened attentively and seemed to care. I did not tell him the over-riding reason for our being treated thus. I doubted that Stand could deal with racism any more honestly than his liberal colleague from the east.

Stand admonished me to try to get along better with my house staff. He, in turn, would see that the student-priests of 9-West were given a more compassionate resident, one who did not shun her responsibility to teach.

"You know, they did see some improvement, recently." He told me as I rose. I shook his hand, then left.

The day had grown colder. The sun cast a tentative yellow beam upon the brown face of the earth, then withdrew from the onslaught of the advancing clouds.

CHAPTER 82

Shelter us from the wrath of your priests.
--unwritten prayer of the student-priests

The seventh week of Medicine found the student-priests of the fellowship of the eye at the V.A. Hospital. Most students disliked the V.A. They preferred the computer printed lab values of the U., the abundance of support staff, and the greatly diminished work load. Many of the students complained also of what they perceived as the unwillingness of the V.A. staff to cooperate with them, and the generalized sluggishness of the V.A. System.

I liked the V.A. I found opportunities there most of my colleagues did not. The increased patient load and the lower ratio of doctors to patients meant more responsibility and a greater chance to both see and do more for the student who was willing to work. Indeed, tests were slow in being performed at the V.A., but true emergencies were done as rapidly as at the U. I had no problems with the staff as did so many of the house staff and my fellow students. I found two keys which worked at the V.A. and anywhere else. First, I spoke to the staff as people entitled to respect. Second, I never expected more than I was willing to give.

The seventh week of Medicine brought other changes, as well. It brought a more sane on-call schedule, every fourth as opposed to every third night. This meant I could occasionally have a social life.

The fellowship of the Saddened Eye was three—Larry, Ron, and I. Reggie, who had suffered greatly for his association with the student-priests of 9-West, was no longer with us. Each of us had received horrible evaluations.

However, it had been arranged from the start that Louis, Ron, and I would complete the twelve weeks of Medicine 1 together. There were only three students to a team at the V.A.

The change in house staff did not afford us the relief for which we had hoped. Things had not gone according to plan. We were to have been assigned Marilyn Savoy, but at the meeting where the selection of residents was announced, another team had requested the popular Savoy. Stand had looked at us and remained silent. We, too, had said nothing. He made the change that the student-priests had requested. Belatedly, through that unswervingly accurate source of information, the student grape vine, we learned that we had been given the worst resident of the lot.

CHAPTER 83

Protect us, our God, as we battle against Cancer, master servant and soldier of Death.
--prayer of the priests of the God of Life

It did not jibe. Before me stood a strong, virile man. His dark skin held a velvety smoothness which bespoke of royalty. In the homeland of his ancestors, my ancestors, he might have been a high lord, a king. I looked again at the card which I had stamped before seeing the patient. The name on my card matched the addressographed band on his wrist. Kurt Bird, my intern, beckoned me to begin my exam. Over the phone, Kurt had said that the man before me, our new patient, had wide-spread lung cancer, that the entire right side of his chest was one large tumor. The oxygen, which ran at an extraordinarily high rate, attested to the man's severe lung disease. Still, he was so strong, such a picture of health, and so young.

Once again, I looked at the card, re-calculating his age. Leon Hardy was fifty-one years old. He looked to be thirty-eight. Fifty-one? I looked at the man before me, noticing that he panted slightly even at rest. His sweat-damped brow emanated an aura of pleading. The man was pleading for air.

I checked the position of the nasal canula. They were properly positioned. The oxygen tank ran at near maximum rates "I already ordered a blood gas on him," Kurt called toward me. He lifted the ear piece to his stethoscope waiting my reply.

"O.K." I answered.

He replaced the ear piece. I placed my black bag on a nearby table and began my examination of our robust-looking charge.

CHAPTER 84

Misery is a creation whose origin is in our hearts.

--the Heretic Priest

Doc, you got a minute?" A tall attractive, well-dressed woman in her late thirties called to me. My work load for the day was normal which meant that I had little time to eat, much less talk, if I wanted to leave at a reasonable hour. She had always been polite, cordial with me as I had seen her several times with the handsome Mr. Hardy. Her quiet stately, proud demeanor belied the constrained desperation I sensed in her voice. I could not ignore her cry.

"Sure..." I beamed a smile her way. "Would you like to sit down?" "Thank you." She folded the full skirt of her printed dress under her in a single gracious movement. She stared absently at the wall in front of her for a moment. A white uniformed figure passed. "Doc, . . ." The words came slowly, only after a struggle. "How is he doing?"

The question was simple enough, appropriate, expected. The answer, however, lay in the realm of deep, unresolved complexities. The answer depended on many issues, but the single most important determinant of my answer was to whom I was speaking. I knew this woman to be a girl friend of my patient. She was the main one, I presumed. The nurses had told me of an incident which had taken place when the woman to whom I spoke and another "friend" of Mr. Hardy had each learned of the other's existence when they had met at the bedside of Mr. Hardy. The woman before me, whose name I did not know, had been often present when the team of priests had spoken with Mr. Hardy. Though Mr. Hardy was my patient whom I had been intimately involved with since his admission, though I knew his case backward and forward, I suspected that there was much she could tell me of his condition which I did not know. My respect of her knowledge of my charge only further confused my answer.

She did not want to hear that Mr. Hardy was a fifty-one year old man with a fifty pack-year history of cigarette smoking who now suffered from wide-spread lung cancer which obliterated one lung and made the other almost totally useless. She was not interested in my polished, well-written write-up of his tragic, but straight forward case, nor did she want a summary of the six-inch stack of papers which comprised his medical record. I did not believe that she wanted to hear what we both knew, that Mr. Hardy was terminal, that no matter what we did, he would still die within weeks. I did not know what it was she was asking, but I knew it was not these.

"We-e-ell, . . ." I paused, searching the ceiling for words. I spoke as gently as honesty would permit. "He seems to be doing OK for the moment." I paused a time watching her expression. Anguish marched in waves across her countenance. It was followed by a painful composure. "But that does not change the underlying disease that he has." I wanted to avoid the word cancer. "There is little we can do about that." I had spoken the naked truth.

"Doctor, you think he would have done better if he had've took that chemotherapy when he first got cancer?" Her protracted, painful expression told me that we were getting to the heart of the matter which had caused her to corner me.

I considered her question. "No." I spoke slowly. "Chances are he would be about the same." The dawn of relief edged her face. "His disease does not respond well to any treatment unless it's caught very early, much earlier than it was when he first came."

She breathed a deep sigh. Her shoulders eased as if relieved of a great burden. "Doctor, when he first found out that he had lung cancer, they tried to get him to take that radiation therapy and chemotherapy and he wouldn't." I recalled a short note to that effect in one of his hospital summaries. There was a space of several months, almost a year, where he had not been followed at the V.A. I had not thought much of this as I had combed his medical records.

"He did not have any money, not much, anyway, and I only got a little. But he wanted to go to this doctor out here in Rushmont who treats cancer with natural medicine. He don't use no regular medicine. He charges a hundred and eighty dollars per injection. He tried that for a few weeks and that didn't seem to do him much good. So, he heard about this health club in Mexico. He went down there. Somewhere on the coast past Sobrino. That cost five-hundred dollars a week. It was a real nice place, though. Everything was from nature. They let me visit him as much as I wanted. They made everything he ate right there, nothing artificial. They had an exercise program to help get all the impurities out your body. But after a few weeks, he wasn't getting no better there either, so he had to come on home when my money gave out. He just stayed at home till he got so he couldn't manage no more. He finally let me bring him here. I prayed for him, but . . ." Water welled within her eyes, she stopped them from splashing headlong onto the floor only with a great effort.

I reached for a handkerchief, on the chance that the will that drove this proud, and now penniless, woman might fail her for one brief moment. It did not. I was grateful as my pockets were as empty as hers.

CHAPTER 85

The interplay between disease and the human psyche make the manifestation of illness varied and unpredictable.

-- a priest of the God of Internal Medicine

I **glanced at my** watch as I stepped from the elevator. My footsteps sounded loudly as I hurried to 3-North. As usual, the temperature sheet, on which the nurses recorded vital signs, was not in its designated place. Louis was coming out of one of the patient rooms. "Seen the heat sheet?" I called out as I peered under notebooks on the desk. "Heat sheet" was the name that Louis had coined for the temperature sheet.

"Here it is. No temps last night." Louis answered.

"Good!" I grabbed one of the surfeit stethoscopes which always hung on the medication carts at the V.A. As I passed his room, I could see Mr. Hardy standing in front of the set of drawers at the side of his bed. Time moved with vicious speed as I urged each of my patients to breathe deeper and faster. Luckily, I was able to check my charges swiftly as there were no abnormalities.

It was Mr. Hardy's turn.

"I got to leave here." Mr. Hardy told me as I laid the still cold stethoscope on his bare chest.

"Don't talk now, O.K.?" I said. "Just breathe deep." Recalling his chest x-ray and listening to his lungs, I was again amazed at how robust the man appeared.

"Doc, I might have to leave here."

"What do you mean?"

"There's somebody trying to cheat me out of some money, trying to take advantage of me while I'm in here." He spoke two or three more sentences to which I only half listened.

"O.K., O.K." I said. "Look, right now I have a couple of things I have to do before rounds. I'll come back after rounds and we'll talk about it. O.K., Mr. Hardy?"

He seemed somewhat calmed by this. "O.K., doc." As I left his room, I remembered that I had not checked the counter for lab slips that the blood drawers could not obtain. As I passed the desk en route to my last few patients, I breathed a sigh of relief. There were no samples for me to draw. I checked the last few patients, quickly, scooped up my white coat, and was present just as the team entered the room of our first patient.

We moved slowly, deliberately, through several rooms. We stopped at the door of a patient who was being treated for tuberculosis just long enough for Kurt to nod in answer as Joel asked complacently, "Status quo?"

The next room the team entered contained four patients. Only one of these was ours. The other occupants of the room wore hurtful, slighted expressions as we gathered around our charge. The chart rack, pushed by the resident, Joel Frye, moved on to the four-bedded room next to the nurse's station.

Mr. Hardy spoke to the resident as we approached his bed. "I'm going to have to get out of here," he declared.

"Why's that, Mr. Hardy?" Joel asked. His tone, as always when he spoke to patients, interns, or students, was condescending.

"I got to go take care of some business."

"Mr. Hardy, you're in no condition to leave the hospital." Joel answered.

"I know, but he came around here this morning."

"Who, Mr. Hardy?" the resident asked.

"He trying to cheat me out of some property. He don't know I know what he's up to. He already come by here this morning."

"We won't let him bother you anymore." Joel placated our charge.

Mr. Hardy settled down into the bed, then peered up at the acoustic-tiled ceiling. A nurse entered the room, stood with the team. "He's up on the roof, right now."

"How do you know he's on the roof?" Joel asked.

"He's right there," he said. pointing upward. Seven sets of eyes rose to the ceiling. Our patient peered at a misplaced piece of acoustic tile. "See that crack move?"

"No, Mr. Hardy. Do *you* see it move?"

"Yeah, right there and he got a gun." He is crazy, I thought. The man has gone mad. The realization hit us all.

We huddled in the hallway. The question was whether the cancer had spread to the brain causing Mr. Hardy's sudden change in behavior or was our charge simply mad? As I wrote out the consultation request to Neurology, I hoped that cancer was the cause of the change for it was something we could treat, at least temporarily. The other possibility was one for which I had little hope.

CHAPTER 86

Grant us courage in the face of adversity.
--a prayer from the House of
the God of Life

It was a quiet night. At ten o'clock all my work was done and there were no admissions pending. I was tired, though, unusually so for such an easy night. The intern was asleep. Unlike me, he did not question good fortune when it arrived, but rather took every benefit it offered. I was too tired to read. Suspecting, as I always did while on call, that an impending disaster waited around every corner, I decided to make one final round before I tried to sleep. I began on the wing which our team shared with another medical team. As I reached the hallway which led to the two pods for which my team was responsible, I saw two nurses and an orderly. standing at a bathroom door. Gladys, one of the nurses, beckoned to me urgently.

"What's the matter?" I asked.

"Mr. Hardy locked himself in the bathroom." Gladys' voice held both concern and annoyance. "He's jammed himself against the door. Maybe you can talk him out." My patient screamed something incoherent.

"Mr. Hardy?" I shouted my patient's name, told him who I was. He shouted something I could not understand. "What?"

"Yeah, I hear you, doc."

"Mr. Hardy, open up the door."

"Doc, I can't."

"Why not, Mr. Hardy?"

"He's out there, doc. He trying to get me." His voice sounded crazed, desperate.

"Who's that, Mr. Hardy?"

"The one with the green shirt." Conviction filled his voice. I turned to Gladys. "Is there anyone around here like that?" Gail, the second nurse, sucked her teeth disgustedly.

"No!" she answered sharply. The other two figures in white uniforms chuckled.

"Mr. Hardy, there's no one here now."

"Yeah, he still there, doc. He waiting in the corner there."

"Mr. Hardy, I'm right here. He can't bother you when I'm here."

"Yes, he can, doc."

I turned to the two nurses and orderly. "Does he have any oxygen in there?"

"There's his oxygen there." Sandra pointed to a transparent green tube lying on the floor.

"Well, then all we have to do is to wait a few minutes. He'll soon pass out without his oxygen."

The three figures looked at me incredulously. Several long minutes passed during which I tried to appear nonchalant. The anxiety rose steadily. There was no sound from the bathroom. What if he's trying to hurt himself, I thought?

"Let's try the door again." The knob turned freely. "I can't push the door open." I said. "He must be pushing against it."

"Wait a minute. Let me help you." Jamie, an orderly from a nearby wing appeared. He moved to put his shoulder to the door.

"Mr. Hardy? . . . Mr. Hardy?" I called. He did not answer.

"He must be out, doc."

"Yeah." We tried to push the door again. As it opened, we could see Mr. Hardy sprawled on the floor. The two nurses, Jamie and I dragged him into the hallway. I was pleased to find that though he was unconscious, he was otherwise alright.

"Hey, doc?" My patient was beginning to wake up.

"Yes?"

"He still here, doc?"

"No, Mr. Hardy, he's gone."

Without warning, my charge became suddenly a writhing ball of flailing arms and legs. The four of us tried vainly to control him.

"You think we should get some help?" Sandra looked at me.

"Well, what do you think?!" I snapped as I caught a flying elbow two inches in front of my face.

She spoke a hurried message into the telephone. The operator's voice came urgently over the loud speaker. "CODE GREEN, THREE-NORTH. CODE GREEN, THREE-NORTH." She repeated the message several times. The four of us struggled with my barrel-chested charge for long minutes.

"Where is everybody?" Sandra moaned.

"I don't know," I answered, "but I sure wish they'd hurry up and get here."

A security guard arrived, followed closely by three men in casual street clothes. One of the men quickly took charge.

"Look out, doc. We got him." He gently nudged me aside. I moved quickly out of the way. Swiftly, with enviable efficiency, they lifted Mr. Hardy onto his bed.

"Got any leather restraints?" the man who took charge asked.

"No." Sandra answered.

"He's going to need them, but give me what you got in the meantime."

Mr. Hardy, though awake, was quiet. I put the oxygen back on him as he was being bound.

"Want to give him anything?" The man who had taken over asked me.

"No," I answered, “not while he's quiet like this”. My patient looked frankly exhausted. He would probably sleep for some time.

I looked for my intern. He was nowhere to be seen. I called Kurt's room.

"Didn't you hear the code green?" I asked the intern. (At the V.A., code green signaled that a patient was out of control and that anyone who was able should respond immediately.)

"I don't go to those things. What are you, *crazy* or something? I'm not getting my head busted."

I told him what had happened.

"I'll come down." he told me.

When Bird arrived five minutes later, I had written both a note in the chart and an incident report. He came, hands in his pockets, peeped in at the patient who was now sleeping, and turned around. "Looks like you got everything under control." The priest sauntered sleepily back toward his on-call room. As he turned the corner, I muttered a long string of curses. The remainder of the night was uneventful. My intern slept the sleep of one innocent and undisturbed. My sweat-drenched patient slept the sleep of one sheltered, temporarily, from harm. I slept the sleep of the exhausted, starting only once or twice as the man in the green shirt flitted past my dreams as he searched for gold and a cure in the House of the God of Life.

CHAPTER 87

Medicine often professes that it is outside the realm of politics. This is not true now, nor has it ever been. Not only is Medicine integrally involved in mainstream politics, but it has its own internal brand of politics which is as aggressive and imbued with intrigue as any on the face of this planet.
--the Heretic Priest

Steele was a tall attending priest. with short, wavy, gray hair whose two eyes, never having learned the concept of mutual cooperation, focused perennially in two completely different directions. To me, the priest, who neared the department chairperson in rank, was an enigma. It was not his distracted vision which puzzled me, nor his manner of looking at his preceptees with but one side of his face, nor his sometimes sullen, quiet moods. What bothered me was something more obvious and yet more subtle than these. Why would a senior attending priest be relegated to precepting medical students, a task usually assigned to fellows and very junior attendings? As I watched the priest with the crooked eye, I sensed, or imagined I sensed, that he too understood the contradiction, the irony, indeed the demeaning nature of the action which placed him before the three student -priests he saw once a week. The obscurity of the priest was pervasive. Though he was well entrenched in the Department of Medicine, neither I, nor most of my classmates, had heard of him before we rotated through Medicine at the V.A. Even the student grape vine was strangely uninformative about the gray-haired priest, admitting, only reluctantly, that he simply was not wanted by the high priests of the God of Internal Medicine, but that as he was tenured and refused to resign, no one could force him to go. It was said that he belonged to another era, another epoch and like the dinosaur had committed the unforgivable sin of failing to adapt. He was given ignominious tasks, such as precepting medical students, with the hope that he would quit. However, tenacity ran deep in his bones.

He held on to his post stubbornly. The student grape vine offered no more information on the shadowed priest. I liked Steele. Louis and Ron liked him, as well. Each of us looked forward to our weekly rounds with the gray-haired priest.

The priest held warmth and a keen sense of humor beyond his surface gruffness. Perhaps because he was one of the few priests who respected us, recognized our intelligence, perhaps because he was, like us, an outcast, we trusted Steele.

It is also possible that it was none of these. Perhaps, as a drowning man grasps at straws, we, feeling both powerless and despised, reached out to the priest with the crooked eye.

We learned a great deal from him and passed many a pleasant hour. He, in turn, learned that contrary to rumor, the student-priests of the Fellowship of the Eye had learned no small amount of Medicine. Once he said this in as many words.

We smiled, hungry for even this left-handed complement.

CHAPTER 88

The role of priest is essentially one of counselor. Though we may lose face in our forays with Death, the patient is the only one who loses life.

--academy lectures

I **spoke my name** clearly into the telephone.

"This is Charise." The woman at the other end of the phone answered. "I just got the gases back on Hardy. They look pretty bad. I called Kurt but he hasn't answered yet and the ambulance is here."

"I'm just around the corner. I'll be right there." I hung up the phone. She was right. Mr. Hardy's arterial blood gases had never been good, but these were the worst yet. The two men wearing identical green pants and white shirt with an emblem watched me impatiently. They were there to transport my patient to the U. for a CAT-scan. We had waited an entire week because time on this new modality was so precious. The University Hospital was one of only two institutions in the entire city to offer the test.

"Those gases are pretty bad." Charise looked over my shoulder as I looked at the lab slip.

"You think it's safe to send him with those gases?" she asked.

"I don't know." I picked up the phone.

"Hey doc, we can't wait any longer. We got other people to transport."

"Just one minute." The paging system cleared. "Kurt?" I identified myself. "Please call me at 5173 regarding Mr. Hardy."

I examined Mr. Hardy's lungs and heart briefly. He had become progressively more lethargic over the preceding eighteen hours. Otherwise, however, he was unchanged.

"Hey, doc, if he can't go now, we'll come back for him."

"When will that be?"

"Tomorrow morning."

"Tomorrow? You can't get back before then?"

"Well maybe in about three or four hours."

I looked at my watch. Mr. Hardy was due for his scan in an hour and a half. People who presented on time often had to wait because of emergency cases. Patients who were late were usually rescheduled a week later.

I paged Kurt again. "Kurt the ambulance is here for Mr. Hardy now, but I need to talk with you right away re- . . ." The allotted time to speak ran out. I drummed my fingers on the table. The ambulance attendant looked at his watch. I paged the resident Joel Frye.

"Doc, sorry. We have to go." They turned to leave." Cursing the intern and resident, I looked at my patient. He did not have a week to wait. If we were to do anything for him, it had to be now.

"Wait!" They turned. "Take him now."

"Somebody's supposed to go with him, right?"

"Yeah." I said. "*I'm* going."

□ □ □ □

The radiologist and CAT-scan technician were eager to teach me the intricacies of their new machine. Though I thirsted for knowledge, my attention was drawn to the sleeping figure on the other side of the glass. With minute intensity, I watched his breathing, starting if it was delayed by the barest fraction of a second.

"You want contrast?" The radiologist spoke to me.

"Huh?"

"Do you want a study with contrast medium?" Puzzlement settled across my face. "What're you looking for?"

"Brain mets."

"We'll do a contrast study."

I paced in front of the glass of the observation room as Mr. Hardy's head disappeared into the massive steel structure of the CAT-scanner. The machine made sounds as if it were the site of an interstellar war. I watched nervously. My patient's breathing was more shallow. I pressed my face against the glass. Protracted minutes passed.

The machine came to a halt. Mr. Hardy was withdrawn from the bowels of the computer controlled x-ray machine.

"He doesn't look so good, huh?' The radiologist spoke to me.

"No, he doesn't."

"What are you?" It was not immediately clear what he meant. " . . a resident, intern?"

"Medical student." He looked at me in mild surprise. My mind stayed on my patient. What should I do for my deteriorating charge? He needed more help than I could give. I did not feel that he should make the trip back to the V.A. without some sort of evaluation and treatment. How could I get help with no member of my team present?

"Maybe you should have someone look at him?"

"Yeah." I answered distractedly. "Where's the phone?"

"Just outside the door, on the wall."

Quickly I dialed the V.A. This time I was able to get through to my resident. I told him of my patient's condition and negative CAT-scan results.

"Get in contact with the Chief Resident. Let him get someone down there to help you."

"O.K." I hung up, called the Chief Resident.

"Call the resident covering the E.R." The Chief Resident told me. In the space of ninety seconds, the E.R. resident arrived. A short man with curly chestnut hair listened attentively as I gave a thirty second synopsis of my patient's course. The resident's pleasantness did not allay my anxiety. The priest listened to my patient's lungs and heart in the hallway.

"I really can't hear much. Let's take him to the E.R. where I can examine him better." The stretcher started into motion. With one hand, I pulled and steered the stretcher. With the other I held an I.V. pole. The resident pushed the rear of the stretcher.

The trip from X-ray to the Emergency Room, only a distance of twenty yards, progressed at a snail's pace in the crowded corridor. As we rounded one of the last turns, the medical resident spoke to me in the same quiet polite tone he might use to say good morning. "I think your patient just stopped breathing."

It could not be. I had checked him only thirty seconds before. I turned. The massive, virile chest, however, was still.

We pushed him quickly over the few remaining feet into the Emergency Room. White coated and green surgical garbed figures came to help. The resident placed a rubber mask with an attached bag over my patient's face, forcing oxygen into his lungs. After a few breaths, the resident removed the mask. My charge showed not even the whisper of an effort to breathe.

"You want us to pump him?" Someone called out.

The resident watched the patient intently for a few more seconds. "No, that's it." The white coats and green surgical scrub suits disengaged Mr. Hardy from the tangle of wires which had sprung upon him, then vanished as quickly, as silently as they had appeared.

Someone drew the curtain, signaling the beginning of the Ceremony of the Newly Dead. I put my emotions in a tightly-bound steel drum as I took part in the ceremonies over my lost charge. Through the distant whirlwind of motions, a voice kept calling, forgive me, forgive me. After a time, I recognized the voice. It was my own.

CHAPTER 89

It's interesting that we deal with illness on a daily basis, and yet handle it so poorly when it strikes us or our families.

--conversation overheard in the House of the God of Life.

Tim was leaving. His mother was very ill. It was not certain that she would live. Tim had been in constant contact with relatives, the doctors caring for his mother. He had known she was doing poorly for some time, but had shared this with his fellow priest-cadets only when he knew that he could delay no more. He had to leave the House of Healing. The tallest student-priest of the Fellowship of the Eye puffed nervously on a cigarette. "You think I should wait till the end of the day?" Tim asked Louis and me.

"No, go now." I told him.

"Yeah, but I hate leaving like this."

"Don't worry about it. Do what you have to do." Louis told him. "You sure?"

"Yes. Go!" I told Tim. The long white coat of Joel Frye floated past the door of the medical student room. He fingered a stack of white index cards in his hand. His appearance on the ward, moving toward D-pod, signaled the beginning of rounds.

"Well, I'll present my new patient and make sure everything is done on him first before I go," Tim told us.

"Tim! The patient's stable. We'll do anything that needs to be done."

"Alright. Thanks a lot."

Rounds proceeded smoothly, complacently, efficiently. Tim presented his patient briefly soon after rounds began. We moved as a milling heard to A-pod to finish rounds. None of the patients Tim followed were on A-pod. I wondered how long he would wait before telling the resident of the emergency in his family. At the times when anguish did not play foremost on his face, impatience was clearly evident. I was impatient for him to begin his trip. It was at least a two hour ride by car to Santa Maria where his mother lay ill.

There were a few more patients to see and discuss, most of whom had been in the hospital for some time, and none of whom were Tim's patients.

"Joel, my mother's very sick." Tim spoke as we moved from a two-bedded to a four-bedded room. The resident did not look at Tim as the student-priest spoke.

"She's in the hospital. She's not doing well. She's not expected to live."

The resident-priest cast a smirk of incredulity at Kurt Bird, the intern, who, in turn, looked at the second intern in smiling disbelief. All this was open, plain to Tim. Hurt cut deep across his face. His brown eyes clouded over. "I have to go to Santa Maria." He was barely able to push the words across his lips. The eyes of Tim's two fellow student-priests shone fire. The priests looked neither at us, nor Tim. Derisive snickers escaped a few lips as Tim waited for a verbal response, some sign that he had the approval of the priests to go. Go, Tim, I thought. Never mind them, just go. Tim, waiting, said nothing. Louis said nothing. The priests said nothing. I said nothing. Finally, Tim spoke. His voice was quiet and uncertain.

"Well, I guess I'll be going now."

"Sure, why not?" Joel Frye waved his hand dismissing Tim with a gesture of insignificance.

"Bye." Tim spoke to the house staff. None of the priests answered. He gathered his belongings quickly. He passed us again as he left.

"Take it easy, man."

"You take care of yourself, now." We called to him.

"O.K." He called back to the two student-priests.

As rounds ended, Louis and I went back to the medical student room. We were not in the mood to talk with the house staff nor share in their chores. Instead, we closed the door and had an hour long discussion about which expletives best described the priests and their unconscionable behavior.

After some time, however, our sense of duty to our patients forced us to look beyond the actions of those entrusted with our education. In the end, it would be the patients who would suffer by our non-cooperation with the house staff.

Ambivalence fitting us closer than our white coats, we went about the business of fighting illness and fulfilling our obligations to our charges and the God of the House of Life.

CHAPTER 90

Every individual is holy. part of that inviolable we call God.

--the Heretic Priest

The only sound was Tim's voice plaintively delivering the history of the present illness. He squirmed uncomfortably in his seat. I sat, my face forming a painfully tight mask of anger. Louis looked at the vice-chairman with thinly veiled chagrin.

The office was large. Its walls were lined with a barely organized array of thick tomes. The desk behind which the chief of service at the V.A. sat was covered with a disordered array of papers. Tim had spent the previous two weeks writing, re-writing; honing his case to a sharp edge. The case, which each student had to present to the chief of service, formed a major part of his/her evaluation. Tim was determined to do well. The priest, an authority in his field who had written a small text which virtually every medical student in the country studied, leaned against the back of his easy chair soundly asleep. His slumber, punctuated by snoring and an occasional head bob, was disturbed momentarily as he asked Tim, for the third time, if the patient had been previously transfused. Tim answered again with a look of quiet dismay.

I suppressed the urge to suck my tongue in disgust. Tim's voice became more feeble. Time passed in an undulating arc, marked only by the nearly broken rhythm of Tim's speech. I paid little attention to what Tim said. I knew the presentation almost as well as Tim. I had heard it many times as the student-priest had practiced on both Louis and me. Seething, I waited time's passing. Tim finished the presentation. Three student-priests waited silently for the priest to awaken. The priest opened his eyes, blinked twice, smiled jovially then began asking questions. As we were already seventy minutes into our allotted hour, the priest was brief.

The door had barely closed to the priest's office when Louis and I let out an unhampered string of expletives. Tim said little, though tears could be seen in the depths of his brown eyes. The tall student-priest clutched his clip board as if he could not determine if he or it might fall. He walked from us deeply sad and dejected. Though we tried diligently, neither Louis nor I could persuade the gentle giant to lift his head back into the clouds where it belonged.

CHAPTER 91

Our struggle is one which may never benefit us personally, but whose value to humanity and the priesthood is immeasurable.
--a priest of the Semi-Secret Order

The mood was down. I joined my two colleagues, members of the Fellowship of the Saddened Eye. I pulled a chair next to Larry whose long legs stretched across most of the small room. It struck me oddly, as it had a few times before, that Louis was tall, fully as tall as I. Somehow it was always surprising to realize this. Tim sat in another corner of the room, looking distractedly at the wall.

"They're going to get us." Louis spoke to me. He swore under his breath. I knew what he spoke of. The subject had occupied much of our thoughts, though we never spoke of it. What would be our evaluation in Medicine 1, the sanguine rite of passage of the priests of the God of Internal Medicine? I held no over-abundance of hope. The priests had been consistent in their distaste for the members of the Fellowship. I passed a time in thought, my head resting on my chest. A half-ray of hope suddenly came to me. "Even they can't be that dumb. They wouldn't flunk all three of us. It would be too obvious what they were doing." Even as I spoke, I realized that my words, instead of bringing encouragement, only confirmed my colleague's prediction of doom.

"Well, maybe *you* might pass . . ." The sentence trailed off. There was no reproach in Louis' voice. Tim issued an assenting hum. I protested feebly, while wondering if they might be right. I could not leave my friends in such a state. The forlorn look, devoid of even a whisper of hope was a pain that I shared with them. I began calmly, logically to explain the possible courses of action of the priests charged with our education in the rites of the God of Internal Medicine. I approached the situation as a simple political exercise as neither my colleagues, nor I, believed that we could trust the humanity of our teachers. If they were to get any of us, they would get all of us, I began. It was obvious from the treatment which we received, that we were viewed as a single entity. They would be hard pressed to justify-their claims of poor performance with no objective evidence to support them. My fellows looked at me doubtfully. I continued. The Standings and Promotion Committee, the committee which would review the actions of the priests of Internal Medicine, had a surprising record of siding with most students who had appeared before it to protest what had been felt to be arbitrary and unjustified decisions by course directors. If we took our case before the Committee, I argued, they would side with us as not passing us could never be justified. The priests of the God of Internal Medicine did not like us, but they were not stupid.

My colleagues looked at me still a bit doubtful, but somewhat more reassured. I was still Keeper of the Flame.

The fire glowed in their eyes.

As I rose to leave the room, I hoped that I had spoken the truth.

CHAPTER 92

Protect us!

--written on a bathroom wall at the Academy of the Priests of the God of Life

Everyone knew before we did. The priests of our team knew, though they gave no indication of their castigation of the students in their charge, as we rounded the following morning. The course directors knew. The attending-priests of the God of Internal Medicine knew. My first knowledge of what had occurred came from that annoyingly accurate information system--the student grape vine. The priests of the God of Internal Medicine had made their final decision. In the end, not the New England liberal with the proud civil rights record, nor the few house staff who took the time to know us, nor the somnolent affability of the vice-chairperson, nor the penetrating gaze of the outcast priest with the crooked eye could save us from the blindness which afflicted the priests who served the God of Internal Medicine.

We did not pass Medicine 1. The entire Fellowship of the Eye was sacrificed on the altar of the God of Internal Medicine.

A few days later I received a letter. It confirmed what I already knew. Further, it set a meeting with the course director in one week.

In the days before the appointed meeting, my mind was subject to a myriad of emotions--disbelief, anger, humiliation, and finally outrage. Fury rose further with the arrival of my scores on the Medicine 1 written examination. The scores were average. Not high, not low, average. The priests of internal medicine did not have a leg on which to stand. Not a single piece of objective evidence--not my write ups, my patient notes, my performance on their exam supported their position.

Strategies began to form. I needed to go to the Standings and Promotions Committee, the academy's final tribunal on matters of student performance. Thoughts equally of retribution and vindication, clearing of my name filled my mind. I needed evidence. Fortunately, I had kept all my write-ups. The priests would supply me with the exam scores.

I needed an advocate. I had no faith in my appointed adviser, a pediatrician whose major field of study was a little known metabolic disease. I knew he could not be depended upon when the going got tough. I needed someone in whom I had full confidence. I needed Garret Frank.

I dialed his number, told Dr. Frank that I needed to talk to him. His only question--was the following afternoon soon enough?

CHAPTER 93

We are often called upon to rise above the many times petty and unwarranted prejudices of the world in which we live. Most often we succeed. However, there are times we do not. We need to be cognizant of these times. We need to grow beyond them for the good of the priesthood and humanity.
--the Heretic Priest

I spoke with Dr. Frank in his office in the Basic Science Building. He considered me calmly through long fingers which were poised before his face as I related events of the preceding twelve weeks. As I was inextricably enmeshed in the tale which caused anger to flow in the retelling, I excused myself several times for being unable to give a totally unemotional account. "Don't worry about that, just tell it the way you see it," he told me each time. His, at once, strong and soothing baritone voice reassured me.

I completed my tale of, then told Frank of my plans to fight the searing injustice, to take my case before the Standings and Promotion Committee. He listened attentively, then asked a few questions. Finally, we turned to my course of action.

"Are you sure that's what you want to do?" He raised his long fingers before his face and raised his eye brow ever so slightly as he asked the question.

I was suddenly alarmed. Was he mad? Of course, I was going to fight this to the very end! "Sure, I'm sure! What do you mean?"

Frank was unflappable. "Is that really the best thing to do."

Doubt began to envelope me. "You don't think I have a good case?"

He leaned toward me. "Don't get me wrong. I'm on your side." Somehow, I needed to hear him say that he believed in my cause. After he said this, I was able to listen to the things he told me. "You'll probably win your case. That's not the issue. It's just that sometimes these things take time."

"What do you mean?"

"Even if you win, and you probably will. It may take six or eight months of wrangling. This coming year you'll be on easy street. Your last year is really downhill. Do you really want that aggravation?"

"You think I should not fight them?"

Frank never told me what I should do. Instead he guided me to my own conclusions. This was one of many tactics which I learned from my talks with the priest-confessor.

"It might be easier for you to just do what they want you to do. “Tell you what, why don't you at least hear what they have to say?"

The fighting spirit within me was strong. I could not surrender before the battle. All I could do then was to agree to consider the priests' offer.

"O.K." I stuttered an answer. "Let me think about it."

The implications of such a prolonged battle began to weigh upon me. Medicine 1 was a prerequisite for several of the electives I - would take in my fourth year. A few of these electives were extremely important to me as I had deemed them necessary to my becoming the doctor that I wanted to be. My medical school training was not over. I was very much aware of my need for further training in several areas. If I won my case, but was prevented from taking these electives because there was not enough time left before graduation, my victory would be a hollow one.

It seemed that the priests of the God of Internal Medicine had out-maneuvered me, no matter which way I turned. I saw visions of the priests holding their sides as the sound of wide-eyed laughter shook them until they were weak.

Garret Frank watched me placidly. As I put up no shield with him, I knew he could trace the lines of my thoughts quite clearly upon my face. I looked into his brown eyes. He was right. He knew it. I knew it.

"Well, let me give it some thought." I rose to leave.

"O.K." He nodded at me, his fingers before his face again.

"Take care." I tried unsuccessfully to flash a brief smile at him.

"O.K."

I had entered Frank's office filled with indignation, ready for a council of war. I left feeling something beyond cornered--I felt crushed. They had won.

I turned to leave the priest-confessor's office. I saw nothing but the gray unwashed floor as I walked slowly toward the stair case.

CHAPTER 94

Ageless and beyond the touch of time,
Hope forever answers all who call.
--a poet-priest

The office, as almost all those in the Basic Science Building, was small, cramped, over-packed. A young woman my own age looked up disdainfully from her typing as I entered, then continued as if I were not there. She sat behind a desk which while only of minimal size was far too large for the sparse space. She took as much care with her medium-length, cherry red nails as she did with the text she was typing. She was the younger of my adviser's two secretaries. The other, a heavy but not obese woman with silver strands highlighting her black hair, always made me feel welcome.

Though I invariably came at the request and convenience of my adviser, the young woman who sat before me indicated always by her actions and expressions that she considered me an unwanted intrusion. She said nothing as I stood before her.

"Excuse me," I told the woman my name. "Would you tell Dr. Frederick that I am here." I could hear my adviser speaking on the phone in the next room.

"Just a minute." she said distractedly. "I'll see if he is in." She looked intently at a portion of the manuscript, then pecked a key.

"Shoot!" She withdrew her finger quickly, examining the nail for any defect. Still looking at the nail, she rose, turned in the narrow space, and entered Frederick's inner office. As I was obliged to stand almost against the door, conversation was overheard easily. She spoke to the priest regarding the thick handful of papers which she had carried into the room with her. He asked her if I had arrived. She answered yes. Why had she had not told him? I had just arrived, she said. My adviser, who was becoming impatient, told the secretary that the papers all could wait. Her hand on the half open door, she turned to ask him about a final correspondence. Annoyed, he told her the proper person to answer the question. She looked into my face as she exited, anger and embarrassment written across her reddened countenance. At another time I might have had a sardonic smile across my face. That morning I simply looked at her with an unmoving equanimity.

"You can go in now."

I thanked her.

My advisor greeted me jovially as usual, smiling broadly at me. I was forced to admit that Frederick was very personable. I felt also that our relationship was strained.

There was a great deal of history which I felt had placed a distance between us over the years (it seemed like centuries) I had been at the Academy. Our meetings, as this one, were always around an academic crisis. There had been a number of times when I needed a strong advocate, when my adviser's support, lukewarm at its best, had vanished altogether in the face of adversity. Though I liked him, I felt that he could not be counted on when the going was tough. It was only because I had admitted that Frank was right, that I would have to strike a bargain with the priests of Internal Medicine, that I allowed Frederick to represent me at all. His role at the meeting was strictly as an observer, a witness against later change to the terms of my further tutelage under the priests of Internal Medicine. Frank had offered to fulfill the role of advocate for me. However, knowing how busy he was and that other students needed his services in cases where his strong advocacy would make a difference, I had declined his offer.

"Ready to go?" Frederick flashed a smile at me. I nodded. I do not remember if I tried to smile back at him. I know that if I did, it was a useless effort. He rose. I followed half a step behind the pleasant priest of the Child God as he walked toward the V.A. hospital. I felt both apprehensive and numbed.

CHAPTER 95

It is humans, not Gods, who quarrel.
--the Heretic Priest

My **awareness of** the present was returning. The numbness, the distance within myself to myself was leaving. I was not going quietly to slaughter. No. I was angry. The depth of my anger surprised me. I will fight them, I thought, with no support if necessary. I was not going to accept their verdict. They were wrong, brazen in their disregard for even a pretense of fairness. No, I calmed myself. Whether they were right or wrong was not the issue. It never had been. The question was how to survive the injustice so that I came through it as whole as possible. No matter how I tried to convince myself to accept what the priests offered, I knew I could not accept just any terms. There had to be, at least, a semblance of fairness. I would not repeat another twelve weeks of Medicine. Beyond this, clouds of uncertainty threatened to engulf me, again. I did not know what I would accept.

Frederick and I were shown into Stand's office. The boyish-looking, gray-haired priest rose to greet us. He extended a hand to Frederick. We sat down. Stand asked if Frederick had seen the evaluations. Frederick had seen them. The priest of the God of Internal Medicine began in a congenial tone to explain that his fellow priests felt that I needed more time in the halls of their God. Stomach churning, I listened. I wondered when he would get to the real meat of the issue--how much time and under what conditions.

Frederick interrupted Stand. The voice of the priest of the God of Children was impatient. "You know, reading those evaluations, I can certainly see where George gets the idea he has been treated unfairly." The priest continued in an annoyed nasal tone. "Reading those evaluations, it's certainly not clear to me what, if anything, he did wrong especially considering that he was getting positive feedback on another level at the same time these people had such negative opinions of him. I don't know about other services, but I get the impression it's the same as on Pediatrics where we deal with students in an altogether different manner. We're much more straightforward. We figure our job is to teach the students and not to make life difficult for them. But I guess that's why different sorts go into different specialties. It sounds to me, from what I can glean of what went on on this rotation, that George ran into a bunch of assholes who really didn't spend the time either teaching or evaluating him the way they should have." Stand's face colored slightly at the last remark.

Had I heard correctly? Was Frederick defending me? Had he actually called the priests of Internal Medicine "assholes"? Thus far I had paid little attention to my adviser. He was present as a witness, nothing more. Stand, whom I had been trying unsuccessfully to read, and whose face had not left my eye sight since I had sat down, was actually the man with all the cards. However, this change in my adviser caused me to turn and face him fully. He continued to deliver a scathing attack on the priests of the God of Internal Medicine. I was very surprised that he was able to see through the facade of the priests, surprised that he actually took up my cause. I had told him only that I had felt that the verdict of the priests was unfair. I had not poured out my heart to him as I had to Frank.

As Frederick spoke, Stand's face became increasingly more crimson. Though I liked Stand, had no animus toward him, I enjoyed seeing him squirm as Frederick told him all the things I had longed to say about the priests who served the God sometimes called "the Flea". Stand tried to smile amicably. Some minutes later, when Frederick had finished his tirade, Stand began to speak.

"This is what we've come up with." He leaned gravely over a sheet of paper which lay on his desk. I turned to face the gray-hired priest. I was filled with waves of anxiety and anticipation. Now was the time, the time when the priests would exact their punishment for the crime seen only in their blindness. How many weeks, how many clerkships would I be forced to give up to fulfill their requirements.

In my mind, I had already given up my ICU sub-internship. A rigorous and much sought after rotation. It was the first of my fourth year. How many others would I be forced to give up as well? Would I be forced to give up my Medicine sub-internship as well? It also was in the beginning of the academic year.

I listened to the gray-haired priest, entranced, weighing every word, every gesture. He spoke several minutes in which I measured time in constricted breaths. " . . . I think you'll find that acceptable." The boyish priest with straight gray hair ended. He looked at me with a half-concealed smile, waiting my reply. I was in a different time than he. I was still evaluating the tape in my mind from several sentences before. Time passed slowly as I arrived at the present. The expectancy in his eyes registered. There was a question in his statement. It was incumbent upon me to reply. I blinked, replayed the tape in my mind.

Had I missed something? Slowly, I evaluated each of his words. As I did so, a leaden fog began to lift. I had been offered four weeks of Medicine sub -internship to fulfill the requirements of the priests. But I was already scheduled to-do a Medicine sub-internship for four weeks. It worked out perfectly!

I could easily shift the four week rotation to the open slot in the final four weeks of my third year. I could take all my fourth year clerkships as planned. It was almost a full minute as I processed Stand's proposal. Oh yes, I should say something.

"That sounds reasonable to me."

"Good." The boyish priest intoned. He made small talk for a moment. As Stand rose and extended his hand to my adviser, his face colored slightly, perhaps in remembrance of the castigation given the priests of his house. I rose.

As I turned to leave, I remembered that I had been warned to get specific goals, specific areas that I was to work on so that this would be the last such meeting I would have with the priests of Internal Medicine. After mentally kicking myself for the oversight, I realized that in a preceptorship type of instruction as that in medicine, efforts to give rigidly specific goals were useless. Frederick and I walked the few hundred yards back to his office largely in silence. I had much to think about. Something bothered me. It was only after several minutes that I was able to discern the cause of my discomfiture. It did not make sense. That was what it was. It did not make sense. The meeting with Stand had been necessitated by the feeling of the priests that I had been unable to perform adequately as a third-year clinical clerk. However, they were saying that I would finish out the time they had added to my third-year rotation not as a student, but as essentially-a priest. (A sub-intern, usually a fourth-year medical students, functioned as an intern. The only differences were that the sub-intern had to have his/her orders co-signed by a resident within twenty-four hours although the orders could be carried out immediately, and the sub-intern usually carried fewer patients. The sub-intern's responsibility to those patients was the same as that of the intern.) How could it be that I had not learned enough medicine to be adequate as a lower-functioning clinical clerk, and yet be promoted to the role of priest?

As Frederick and I walked through the weed-cluttered group of shacks which remained from the time when the campus had been a military base, I reflected upon my meeting with the gray-haired priest of Internal Medicine. What had prompted this semblance of fairness by priests who had dealt so unfairly with me for twelve weeks? Did they have a conscience after all? Was it possible that they were not as blind as the unseeing eyes of Boford and Steele implied, or did they fear that their case would fail before the Standings and Promotions Committee? I did not know. We arrived at Frederick's office. Out of my new found respect and regard for the priest I stayed a few minutes to make small talk. He smiled as he took my hand as I was leaving. I found the strength to smile back.

I thought of going to see Frank, but I had too much thinking to do. My thoughts returned to the priests of Internal Medicine. Had they not won in the end? Had they not humiliated me? Had they not cast aspersions upon my long hours of toil, defamed my best efforts, slandered the Fellowship of the Eye and through us an entire race? Had they not won? Yet, had I not won? Was I not spending exactly the same amount of time under the tutelage of the priests of Internal Medicine as I had planned from the beginning? Was I not spending that time as a sub-intern as I had wanted? Was I not going forward, progressing in level of function, level of responsibility as was right, just? Had I not won?

As I wandered over a grass-covered knoll which sprouted newly-green blades against a sea of pale brown, I realized that though I should see a thousand winters, I would never know who had really won. Truly, beyond the injury to my pride, which would heal with time, it did not matter.

In the end I was the judge that mattered. My own appraisal of me would have to sustain me through the time ahead. Through the fire, I had reached a milestone, had transcended to a higher level. I no longer cared what the priests thought of me. It was only then, as I stood in the sea of speckled grass, that I began to feel at a gut level what I had known intellectually for nearly two years--the only opinion that mattered was the one I held of me.

It was a frightening feeling. It was a deep-down good feeling. A rabbit skittered before me as I started my car.

As the medical school passed out of view, I noticed the impending greenness of the dawning spring.

CHAPTER 96

Without the nervous system, purposeful action cannot take place, volition itself becomes impossible.

Introductory Academy Lectures on the human nervous system

Around me, my colleagues chatted amicably. We were gathered for the first day orientation of the Psychiatry and Neurology rotations. Fortune shined brightly upon me. There was room for two students at Loeb, the outpatient psychiatric institute associated with the academy. Only one student other than I wanted to be placed there. As it was not hospital based and as it required longer hours, it was not very popular.

To the contrary, the outpatient Neurology rotation was a highly coveted gem. The only alternative to outpatient Neurology was four weeks of Neurology hospital wards. Virtually every student I had spoken to thought of time spent there as a prolonged drudgery of rounds on unchanging stroke victims who, most often, were totally unaware of their surroundings and who benefited little from the services proffered them. Most of the students wanted the out-patient rotation. Each quarter a lottery was held to see who would get this very desirablespot.

The chatter of my classmates quieted as the slightly rotund priest, whom I was toknow verywell, placed three scraps of paper on the table before him. The three pieces of paper contained the names of the student-priests who had won the lottery for outpatient neurology. The second name caused elation to rise within me--it wasmine.

Chatter rose again, amicably. Most of the student-priests present, as I, had just finished Medicine 1 and were glad to be released from the lash of the God of Internal Medicine. I relaxed a little. My time under the Twin Gods, Neurology and Psychiatry, promised to be a pleasant one.

□ □ □ □

I arrived at the U. a few minutes after eight o'clock. The shining new outpatient building was almost empty. I approached a security guard, a young man with wavy, raven-black hair and handsome features, I asked where might I find Neurology, Politely, he directed me to a large suite on the second floor. There were several doors in the section of the building occupied by Neurology. Most were locked, I found one open. The inside hallway was deserted. I followed the sound of footsteps. A small woman in a crisp white uniform looked up as I approached, she was in her mid-forties. Her eyes, the color of deeply stained walnut, were friendly.

"May I help you?" It was actually a question not the usual challenge thrust at an intruder.

I told her my name, told her that I was the student assigned to Neurology.

She extended a hand across the counter. "Hi, George. I'm Elena. I'm the head nurse."

" Pleased to meet you." I told her.

She smiled. "There's no one else here now, I usually like to come in early. It gives me a little time to relax before the day begins. Can I get you anything?"

"No, thank you."

"I guess you'll be working mainly with Dr. Karman and he's not in now. Most of the students really like this clerkship."

" So, I 'm told,"

"You'll like it here, too. I'm sure," she continued talking, easily carrying most of the conversation. We spoke for a few more minutes. Other members of the staff arrived.

The noisy clatter of a door being unlocked announced the arrival of Doctor Karman. We were introduced. He carried a bundle of papers and a worn chestnut brief case under his arm.

"Hi. I'll be with you in a minute, George."

"Do you need some help?" He seemed to be having trouble opening the door to his office.

"No, I 'm just fine, thanks. I'm used to doing it this way." He was barely able to talk as he carried a parcel under his chin which he struggled not to drop. The door eased open.

"Just give me a minute to arrange a few things and to make a quick phone call and I'll be right with you."

"Sure" I said. He placed multiple objects on his desk in an orderly fashion. He opened one of the files, reading intently. I watched him a few seconds from outside his door. He reached for the phone. I turned, returning to the nurse's station where already the day's activity had begun.

I returned to Karman's office after a few minutes. He sat reading correspondence. He looked up as I approached. " I didn't mean for you to leave." The priest with kindly brown eyes showed hurt. " I was expecting you to sit down in here while I made the call. It only took a second."

"Oh." I could think of nothing else to say. He smiled warmly at me. "Let's go into the library. It's much less junky in there." He took me through a second door. The library was a long elegant room in which off-white drapes ran from ceiling to floor and allowed a softened sunlight to spill onto the orange-red carpet. A Masonite veneered table with the appearance of the deepest walnut finish ran the length of the room. There were only a few books, only enough to cover the narrow wall at the end of the room nearest Karman's office. The room was obviously used more as a conference room rather than a true library.

He closed the door. "Have a seat," the priest said after he saw that I was still standing, still ill at ease. The priest sat next to me. He delineated my duties on the rotation. There was a genuine warmth in the priest which was undeniable.

I was expected to be at the clinic Monday through Friday from nine until four or five depending upon when the clinic ended. Every morning and afternoon, I would do a complete neurological history and physical on a new patient. This had two purposes. The first--to allow me to sharpen my neurological exam. Secondly it allowed me to be part of the initial evaluation and treatment plan. After I did my history and physical and presented them to the attending of the day, I would accompany the attending the remainder of the session.

"Do you have any questions?" The attending-priest with curly sienna hair and black framed glasses looked at me. I liked the priest. Despite my initial mistrust born of experiences outside the House of Neurology, I liked him.

"No," I answered. I had no questions of the priest that would not be answered with time. This priest, who served the dichotomized God of Neurology, was approachable, human. The priest who reached out and touched a part of me was kind. Yes, that was the word, kind. He put me to work right away. I found the work exacting, stimulating, challenging. I was rewarded for my hard work with things I had forgotten over the previous twelve weeks—teaching, praise, respect. The priests of the God of Neurology respected my judgment and I listened, drank of their wisdom, and respected them. Time passed quickly and pleasantly under their tutelage.

CHAPTER 97

The twin Gods of Neurology and Psychiatry have not always been separate. They were once worshiped as a single entity.

Time has revealed these are often similar, but distinct, entities. Just as once we priests believed that the seat of reason, was the heart, we mistakenly believed that purposeful action and the formulation of purposeful action were one in the same. We realize our error now.

Generally speaking, the formulation of, and initiation of purposeful action, volition, if you will, properly belongs in the realm of Psychiatry. Likewise, the organization and specific workings of the body's sensory and motor functions properly belong to Neurology.

--academy lectures on the Dichotomized Gods, Psychiatry and Neurology

The complete neurological exam on my initial patient of the afternoon seemed to be taking an extraordinarily long time. The patient had too many small, seemingly inconsistent, findings. I had learned from the priests of Neurology that this was to be expected to some extent. However, that if a finding was real it would neither disappear nor show much change with retesting. My neurological history, and physicals, and write-ups which had gone from an hour and a half to forty-five minutes, as I had gained proficiency, was dragging to the end of its second hour with this difficult patient as I made my third trip out of the exam room to get another instrument, my eyes again, ran across the face of the angry patient who sat outside the exam room used by the day's attending. The neurologist of the day was Margie McClung. She was one of the youngest of the attending-priests in the Department, and like all the priests in Neurology, quite bright. Her particular field of interest was seizure disorders. Though, liked by all, she was particularly popular among adolescent patients and medical students. As the clinic was very busy that afternoon, I had little chance to see or talk with the attending-priest until we were half way into the session. I presented my first case to her as well as my findings. I was surprised that she took my exam at face value, repeating a very brief physical only to confirm my major findings. It took time for me to grow used to confidence in the quality of my work by my supervising priests. Though pushed for time, she took me aside and went over the anatomical explanation of my physical finding. Quickly, we both dove into the waiting back log of patients.

After a time, the attending priest called me to her exam room. As I entered the exam room. I saw the angry patient. Dr. McClung introduced me to her.

“Hel1o," I said.

"Hi!" As the woman spoke, a sincere smile dispelled the angry mask she wore. I was surprised at the immediate change in her expression. The attending physician saw the look of surprise on my face and smiled. "Looked like she was angry, didn’t she?"

"Yes, " I nodded.

"Mrs., Patrick often looks that way. She has Parkinsonism."

"My friends a1ways tell me I look angry. And I can be in such a good mood." The woman chuckled.

We chatted for a few minutes more before seeing the last few patients in clinic. I marveled at how I had been so completely mistaken. It was only the first of several times I would mistake the faces of the divided God. As I learned so very much under the tutelage of the priests of Neurology. Experiences such as these served to keep the confidence of one priest-cadet within reasonable limits.

CHAPTER 98

Neurological diseases have virtually all the hallmarks of psychiatric illness.
At times, even those well versed in both fields find the distinguishing between the two almost impossible.

--academy lectures, on the Twin Gods Neurology and Psychiatry

The afternoon was passing quickly, too quickly. Though I hurried, my work was taking a long time. I left the examination room for the second time, I noticed a forty-ish, rather plump woman whose expression seemed to grow more irate each time I passed her. I hoped that she fell to the attending.

The light shined upon the pink inner surface of the young girl's mouth.

"Open your mouth wider, please,"

"Huh?" She answered in an annoying nasal tone.

"Open your mouth wider." I spoke louder, trying not to let my growing impatience show in my voice. "You can close it again." I was satisfied that the movement in the back of her throat was indeed normal, that what had appeared abnormal initially was the result of poor effort on the part of my young patient. I strained to keep my face in a non-committal grimace of neutrality, as the girl's mother looked on, agreeably.

There was a knock at the door. My chagrin rose to a peak as the attending priest of the day, a strong -framed woman about forty years of age, entered the room. Her brown hair fell in crisp, even lines across, her forehead and the back of her neck. "How's it going?" she asked. Her manner told me she was anxious to see the patient.

"I haven't got anywhere near finished." I admitted guiltily•

"That's OK." She smiled pleasantly. "What do you think so far?"

"We-e-ell • • " I began.I felt that the weakness I had observed was inconstant and did not fit well into any neurological syndrome I could recall. I felt that my findings were therefore not "real", that they were the result of less than full effort. I fumbled for the right words, the correct phrases in doctorese which allowed Martha Silverman to understand me, but not the patient or her mother. "There is a question of some weakness in some of the facial nerves. However, the exam is somewhat variable and I'm notsure...."

"Charlotte has myasthenia gravis." The attending priest interrupted. The name of the disease called a cascade of information about an illness studied in great detail by students of the priesthood because of the physiologic principles it demonstrated. It was a disease rarely encountered in clinical practice. I had never seen a patient with the illness.

"Charlotte gets worse as the day progresses." Dr. Silverman spoke to me. I looked at the girl's mother. She looked at me knowingly. Though there was no malice in the woman's face, I felt no small amount of embarrassment.

The woman spoke to me. "We took Christine to lots of doctors before we came here, No one knew what was wrong with her. Finally, we took her to see Dr, Silverman. She was the one who found out what was wrong with her." The woman's face beamed unadulterated gratitude at the attending priest, Martha Silverman said nothing for a moment, only smiled modestly, as if embarrassed by the mother's display of thankfulness and respect. My professor's lectures in my first year at the academy, had left me with the impression that she was reasonably pleasant, but aloof and cool. However, observing her with patients, watching her banter playfully with staff, seeing how she always went out of her way to see that I learned, showed me a warm side of the priest that I had not suspected.

"Myasthenia is difficult to diagnose. The signs are very vague. Most often the diagnosis is missed the first time around. Many of these patients are referred to psychiatrists." For a moment, I wondered if the priest had read my mind.

"Notice Charlotte's nasal tone?" The priest continued,

"Yes."

"She doesn't always talk like that. It gets worse late in the day. Her mother had told me this also, but I didn't know what to make of it, It's one of the manifestations of her disease. The muscles of the pharynx get progressively weaker with use." Understanding began to dawn upon me." It's difficult to differentiate many of the subtle signs from poor effort."

"Are there any specific tests that you can use to differentiate myasthenia from poor effort?"

"Mostly it's just judgment. But let me show you this" Silverman stepped in front of the patient. "Close your eyes, hon"' The girl closed her eyes. "Tight, honey." Wrinkles formed in the girl's eyelids. "See how easily I can open her lids?" The priest spoke to me.

"Yes."

"You notice how her eyes go up?"

"Yes."

"That's called Bell's sign" She said.

"It shows maximal effort." The priest turned to look 'at me. "O.K.?" I nodded ascent.

She turned to the child's mother. "How's Charlotte, doing today?"

"She's been pretty good lately." Small talk continued for several minutes. I stood by quietly.

As I said good-bye, I smiled, grateful that another pearl from the Twin Gods, another jewel from the God of Life and Healing had been given to me.

CHAPTER 99

The dichotomized Gods are still mainly a mystery to us. Psychiatry is still mainly a "Black Box" about which we have a multitude of hypotheses which are workable to varying degrees with regard to minor mental dysfunction and which are virtually useless in defining major mental dysfunction. Likewise, in Neurology we have a myriad of minutia which gives us little notion of the workings of the whole organism. Just as at one time we found it convenient to separate the two Gods, I wonder might not our growing knowledge of the two disciplines, particularly Neurology, cause us to realize that Psychiatry and Neurology are but two faces of the same coin. I wonder, might not our growing knowledge cause us to rejoin the Dichotomized Gods.

--A visionary priest of the Dichotomized Gods

THE THIRD YEAR

You shouldn't have much trouble with this one at all." I sat across the large desk from the benevolent priest, Karman. At least he had always *seemed* benevolent. He smiled at me as he continued. "His daughter brings him to you saying that he seems unable to remember anything, that he can't complete even small tasks, that normally he completes easily. He seems irritable over the last several weeks. Karman continued in detail his portrait of a highly functioning sixty year old businessman who progressively deteriorates over the course of a few weeks. I listened carefully, absorbing every small piece of information. As the priest finished, he looked at me expectantly. I blinked back at him, surprised that the story had ended.

"Well, doctor, what do you think is going on?" I replayed the tale in my mind. I asked a few questions, replayed the tale once more, looking for any hidden traps, subtle pitfalls. My colleagues had all said that this exam was a very difficult one. Fearful of this information obtained through the student grapevine, I had spent much of the previous night's studying some of the more obscure syndromes I had encountered in my four weeks in the House of the God of Neurology. The list of diseases one had to consider for even the more common entities was astounding in length. I had spent less time with the more routine illnesses as I felt confident handling them from my having seen them daily. The bearded priest stirred as he eyed me across the desk which was clear for the first time in my recollection.

"We-e-11." I tried to put off answering the question put to me. The presentation and the answer seemed altogether straightforward, easy.I looked again at the priest.

He did not seem to be trying to trick me. However, with the memory of Medicine 1 still fresh in my mind, I was unwilling to trust the apparent, obvious answer.

I began to become impatient with myself. I had applied myself. I had worked diligently in the House of the priest's God.

I approached the case from a roundabout angle so that I might discuss briefly less likely, but still possible, diagnoses. I saved the two most likely diagnoses for last. My articulate and coherent

presentation surprised me. The priest watched me non-committedly until my conclusion. "It would seem then, from the history and the exam you have given me, that the patient most likely has a slow-growing brain tumor in the left frontal region. However, a chronic subdural hematoma cannot be ruled out."
The priest's eyes lit up. "Excellent! Excellent!" He smiled broadly at me. "You've answered just about all the questions that Iwas going to ask you." I smiled. Still, I was not at ease. Thepriest asked a few minor questions which I answeredwithout hesitation.
Hisexpressionchanged. His facebecame serious. He looked down athis desk ashe spoketo me.Here comes the real test, Ithought.He askedme a question regarding the treatment of a neurological syndrome. He looked up at me, leaning back in his chair. From his pointed, penetrating gaze, it was clear that the priest expected me to have a great deal of difficulty answering the question. I thought the question over only briefly before plunging into the answer. I discussed several treatment modalities, enumerating the risks and benefits of each. The priest was impressed. I had passed the test of fire.
"Thank you," I smiled.
"That's it. You really did good on that."
The priest's face became serious once more. "Now, I'd like to have your thoughts on the rotation and the faculty."
It was clear that the priest was sincere. Also, as I knew some of the history of the medical school, I knew that the Department of Neurology had a tradition of being sensitive to student feedback. I considered my answer well. It was an excellent rotation. I told him. The faculty were excellent teachers. I would recommend the course to anyone. I spoke truthfully to the priest who had dealt with me so honestly for the four weeks I was under his tutelage.
“What field are you thinking about going into?
" I don't know for certain." I answered the priest. "Well, we are very pleased with your work. I discussed it with several of the other faculty members as well. We would be very pleased if you chose Neurology. We'd love to have you here."

I looked across at the bearded, kindly priest. I did not know what to say. I was filled with appreciation and many other good feelings.

"Thank you" I managed to utter through a choked voice.

The priest smiled.

CHAPTER 100

The term schizophrenia denotes in its most severe form, a profound state of dysfunction. It is to schizophrenia that laymen usually refer when they use the term "crazy".

—academy lectures psychotic disorders

The rhythmic clicking of the ball bearings came to a halt as I entered the parking lot of Loeb Institute. I extended the kick stand of my red, three-speed bicycle. The five minute ride from my house had been enjoyable. Though the outpatient facility of the Psychiatry Department was only a mile from my house, I had never been to Loeb before starting my clerkship.

From the layout of the grounds I surmised that the older single-storied, yellow brick building was the focal point of activity. As I passed to the front of it, peering into mildly dusty windows, I saw only one or two people. A newer structure, built in the style of a small office building sat on the main street. Over its gray stone facade hung the name of the man for which the facility was named. I wondered what great works he had performed or money had he contributed to the academy to receive such an honor. The front of the newer building was crisply trimmed, immaculate.

I pushed open the double-door, careful to touch only the metal door handle, careful not to mar the door's mirror finish. A freshly scrubbed and manicured receptionist, Samantha, greeted me pleasantly as I entered. I was beginning to feel that the Loeb Institute which I was in, was not the institute which had been described to me. No one had mentioned the plushness of the office before me nor the calm controlled atmosphere.

When I told the receptionist who I was, she informed me that I was early, that most people had not come to work yet, that I might find Janie, the head therapist, in her office. She directed me to the larger, painted yellow brick building which I had passed moments before

□ □ □ □

Janie was in her office. I looked into a long angular face which seemed held in a moment of perpetual honesty and basic goodness. She rose, smiled, and took my hand as I introduced myself. She gave me a brief introduction to the Institute, told me of the day's planned activitiesbeforeintroducing me tootherstaff members.

"You won't need that." She told me. I looked at her questioningly. "The coat. " She pointed to my white lab jacket.

"Oh." I said•

"You can just leave it in here for now." I placed the coat across the top of a bookcase. She locked the door to her office.

I was introduced to the other four therapists who, with Janie, ran the day treatment program. The first activity of the day was a staff meeting. As the meeting began, my colleague, the second student-priest assigned to Loeb, arrived. Michael Ching was six-feet tall and wore wire-rimmed glasses. Though we had seen one another many times before, we had never had any direct contact. I grew to like the tall student-priest.

Mike and I sat quietly at the end of the long table, listening attentively to what the therapists said. Several times during the meeting a therapist politely, but firmly, asked one of the patients to wait outside until the meeting was finished. It seemed almost a game where the patients (referred to always as "clients" by the therapists) tested how far they could go before being called back. I was assigned to Dawn, a registered nurse, whose soft-spoken empathetic ways contrasted sharply with her powerful build.

After half an hour, the patients were allowed into the large central room where I was to spend most of my time while at Loeb. As the patients entered, I was impressed with how "normal" most of them appeared. I had had visions of screaming, unkempt men and woman. I saw none. Instead, I saw a surprisingly "normal" appearing group of individuals.

I watched the patients closely for a moment then followed Dawn and a patient into her office to observe my first one on one interview.

CHAPTER 101

The introduction of potent medications to control the hallucinations of schizophrenia haled to th virtual disappearancef the "raving maniac". It has placed many persons afflicted with this disease into an ordered and productive life style. However, there still remain those afflicted who go on to follow a progressive and, at present, unalterable down-hill course

—academy lectures on mental illness

The young woman, Jane, followed me into Dawn's office. She smiled pleasantly, l had had been at Loeb for one week and was already performing interviews on my own.

"Please sit down," I indicated a comfortable chair in front of the desk. The woman seated herself, smiling at me again. There was no mistaking the inviting twinkle in her eye. I smiled back at her, pleasantly, soberly, I explained the nature of the intake interview, that my purpose was only to gather data on which to base future treatment. From my training in the first and second year, I had gained adegree of comfort with the psychiatric interview. The free-flowing, almost structureless manner of the psychiatric history suited me well. If one was just the least bit clever, one could get all the information which was needed, yet allow an of conversation.

I began the interview with biological data—age, occupation, marital status. My patient was an employee of the local telephone company. Several weeks before her referral to Loeb, her work had begun to deteriorate. Her work, which was initially quite good, worsened till at the end of each work day she was getting nothing accomplished at all. Also, her supervisor noted that she was acting "strangely."

Finally, the supervisor, whom Jane counted among her few friends, had convinced her to seek treatment for her emotional state.

Something was not quite right. I realized as I listened to my patient that I was getting little specifics as to the exact nature of her dysfunction and that a precipitating event was missing. I questioned my charge more closely, directing the conversation tightly for a short time. She mentioned aparty given bystrangerswhom she thought of as "weird"

"Tell me about the party."

"I didn't know nobody there."

"How did you find out about it?"

"A guy in my building gaveit."

"A friend of yours?" Friends seemed scarce in the little Ihad learned of her life, Perhaps, here was one she had not mentioned previously.

"Imet him by the pool and he invited me to this party."

"Go on, tell me about theparty."

"There was a bunch of people chanting and stuff." She looked at me tentatively, then continued. "They believed in witchcraft and stuff. It wasn't really a party. It was really a meeting of people who believe in magic and witchcraft."

A blue-jean clad figure caught my eye as the young telephone worker spoke, Outside the closed window, standing before a palm in the courtyard, was Sharon, a young schizophrenic in her early twenties who had recently come to Loeb. From where I sat, she stood in almost a direct line of vision with the patient I was interviewing. Sharon stood before the tree, giving it, and the shrubs before her, her total and unwilling attention. Her eyes darted in the chaotic rhythm of a conversation, hallucinations, which only she could hear.

Even the vegetation remained mutely still, oblivious to the murmurings inside the woman's mind.

"There was this man there." I forced my attention back to Jane, the woman inside the room with me, the one whom I was interviewing She spoke of the party, a mysterious man whom she had met at the gathering. "He was the leader of the group. He put me in a trance."

"A trance?"

"Yes. He hypnotized me. He took me back in time to when I was a child. Then he let me play with my powers

"Powers?"

"Yes. He showed me I was the Chosen One, the Christ-Child. Then a star came down." Her face shone with the glaring light of delusional zeal. I had thought before that I had seen a glimmer, but I knew, as she related her experience at the party, that my patient was a schizophrenic. "And it told the people that I was the Chosen One." She continued. "It showed me all the things I had done. And it made me see how when I was a baby how the people worshiped me. I saw how all the people prayed to me because I was Jesus Christ. Then I saw my nephew. I could see into the future when he would have the powers because he was the Chosen One." She was obviously not bothered by the inconsistencies of her beliefs. She wore an expression of supreme self-satisfaction.

I did not know what she referred to regarding the rain.

"Rain?" I questioned.

"Yeah, all the rain a month ago." About three weeks before most of the country had had record-breaking deluges. She continued, her speech only slightly less pressured than previously.

"I made my sister have a boy. I knew she was going to have a boy before she even had him. I said exactly when he would be born. And I made "Saturday Night Fever " go from "R" to "PG". She leaned back and smiled at me proudly.

Outside, Sharon cowered under the pressure of voices, menacing and merciless, which fought within her head.The battle in her mind spilled over into pain-laden tears.

Sobbing racked her body in thunderous waves, I felt an overpowering urge to run outside and hold her, to reassure her,to tell her that the voices, though frightening, could not harm her. I knew I could do none of these.

I returned my gaze to the woman inside who sat before me, legs crossed. "Go on." I urged. She smiled a smile at once seductive and triumphant. I wondered would she be smiling if she knew that probably a life like Sharon's, one filled with painful and increasingly intrusive apparitions, a life where nightmares reigned over waking reality and sleep offered no respite, lay ahead of her.

After a moment, her smile faded. "Then the trance was over. I was back." She was suddenly sad. Finality filled her voice. Her brown eyes flitted restively over the floor. "I missed my powers. I wanted to play with them again." There was silence for a time.The allotted hour was nearly over. We had covered enough ground for an initial interview.

I had learned from Dr. Frank not to end a contact with wounds open. I could feel my patient's gaping hurts. Her powers had been real to her, if only for a brief moment. Their loss was painful. Without them she was simply a socially isolated young woman, undistinguished and ordinary, fragile and afraid. I brought the conversation around to a pleasant topic. She had smiled when she had mentioned her nephew.

"You like your sister's son,don't you?"

"Yes." She smiled.

With a little prompting, she spoke openly of her affection for thebaby boy who was the first grandchild of the family. Several minutes passedin which shebecame more andmoreanimated

We rose to leave. "You live near here?" She asked me.

She stood close, almost touching me as she spoke. The seductiveness had crept back intoher voice and manner

"Not far."

She smiled invitingly as she named severalnear-by areas. She asked if I lived in any of them.

"I live near here." I remained purposely vague. "So, you'l l be joining us on Thursday, right?" I tried to steer the conversation to another subject. I opened the door.

"Yes." We ambled into the main room of the day treatment area. "Will you be here of Thursday?"

"Yes, I'll be here," I scanned the large room. A few people stood about, mainly patients preparing to go to lunch, I did not see Sharon.

"You going to eat lunch now?" my patient asked.

"No, not now".

"Well, maybe we be we could gettogether sometime, huh?" The smile,theonewith theunmistakable invitation was there.

" I'm sure I'll see you here whenyou start."

My patient seemed persistent and unwilling to leave. I was worried about Sharon. "Well, I'm sure you must be starved and I have things I must do."

"Yeah, I guess you must be busy, huh?"

"Yes•" Inodded.

"Guess, I vbetter be going. I'll see you, O.K? She smiled once more as shewaved good-bye. Iwas the first of severalmales, staff andpatients, to bethetargetofher seductive behavior,

Sharon was nowhere in the Institute. Though it was lunch time, I was not particularly hungry. I thought of the two young women. How cruel a lot the fates had given them. They were afflicted with a disease which invaded the privacy of their thoughts, made their senses unreliable. The schizophrenic could not be sure of any object, any voice, any person. Their world was one which had no respected rules, no boundaries, and, far too often it seemed, no escape.

As Loeb gave me my first, in depth, look at the disease called schizophrenia, I found a small amount of comfort in knowing that I was but a passing sojourner in the land of those so afflicted.

CHAPTER 102

It is because of a highly evolved intellect that humans are the Earth's dominant species. This intellect is the key to our survival. Ironically, it is also the only source of knowingly self-destructive behavior of any of Earth's life forms

—academy lectures, self-destruction and the human mind

Rockledge Mental Health Facility. The name conjured up images of patients raging in armless white strait jackets, diets of feces and urine, unrestrained chaos. Though it was part of the University Hospital complex, it was treated as an unwanted step-child, an unwholesome, wished-forgotten family disgrace, tolerated only because it was necessary for the protection of the community and the teaching of the priests of the Dichotomized Gods.

As part of our psychiatry rotation, we were required to spend three evenings at Rockledge. Though I had passed the low-lying brick building a few hundred times, I did not know how to enter it.

I chained the front wheel of my bicycle to the rack.I peered into the dust covered window beside a doorway as I tapped for several minutes. I could hear voices inside. No one answered my knocking. I walked around the fenced yard where I had often seen patients exercising.A gate led to what looked like an ambulance port. I tapped on a heavy metal door. Through the doorsglass, I could see a large bare room with a low, wooden bench bolted to the wall. Another bench ran the length of the room and was also bolted down. The door remained closed. I turned the knob. I was surprised to find that it opened easily. The room had a cold unfriendliness about it. It looked as a rampart taking an uneasy breath before the next onslaught. Distantly, voices could be heard. A figure passed before a grilled window which gave the only view to the inside of the building.

"Hello!" I shouted. The figure was gone before I spoke. I went up to the window. "Hello!" No one answered. I tapped on the window. The thick glass made little sound• I pounded the grating with my fist. "Hello, Hello!"

A button was on the wall next to the window, I pushed it. A high-pitched ringing sounded somewhere beyond the window.

A small figure, wearing a blue and white stripedshirt
and faded blue-jeans appeared on the other side of the heavy metal wiringHe looked at me suspiciously.

"May I help you?" He challenged. I told him who I was, that I was assigned to Rockledge for the evening. He scrutinized me carefully for several more seconds. "The door is over there." He pointed tohis left. Hishands went under the counter as the buzzer of the electronic lock sounded.

□ □ □ □

"Doctor Manor, this is the medical student who is here with us tonight." The small man who had admitted me to the brick fortress told the priest my name. Manor was a slight man with graying blondish hair.

"Hello, doctor." He leaned over the desk and extended a nervous hand toward me.

"Hello, Dr. Manor." I took his hand.

"See you." The small man in blue jeans called. as he exited the room.

"Thank you," I called to his disappearing back.

As I sat, a non-stop barrage of conversation began. The priest spoke almost without pause for breath. He presented the case of a patient whom he had just interviewed, He presented the case in the minute detail that a student might use but not a fully-fledged priest. He arrived finally at the diagnosis he had given the patient. As a way of showing the priest that I understood some basics of psychiatry, I mentioned a second diagnosis which had to be considered in the patient we had discussed, but which was clearly unlikely.

"You know you're right, that *is* a possibility," he told me. I was shocked when the crossed-out his own assessment and put instead, the second, less likely, diagnosis to which I had alluded.

□ □ □ □

A small woman sat in the gray room through which I had first entered Rockledge. She looked about her expectantly. I pushed open the heavy metal door. The woman watched me appraising as I approached. Her black hair was uncombed and matted down in some places, and in others sticking up in a frenzy of unruliness. The printed shift, her single piece of clothing showed most of her left breast through a large rent at the collar. Despite her crazed stare and her disheveled appearance there was an undeniable dignity in her bearing.

She had arrived in hand cuffs. The only history I had was that she had been brought in by the police, screaming, angry, kicking, after taking off her clothes in the middle of an apartment complex.

I told the woman my name. She looked closely, questioningly for some time before she told me of the events that had caused her to come to Rockledge.

"I got powers of healing, you know? "She watched me closely as she spoke. Her words were crisply enunciated.

"Do you really?" I asked calmly, surveying the unkempt person before me.

"Yes. My daughter has the power also. You see, I'm a meta -physician. Not a physician, but a META-physician."

"Oh?"

"Yes. A meta-physician is higher than a physician."
Despite the clearly manifested fringes of madness in her manner, she spoke these words with such conviction that I was forced to steal a glance at my name tag. I was relieved to see that it did not contain the letters "M.D." In the presence of this woman, the priesthood seeme1d truly an ignominious calling.

We talked for a while longer before I returned behind the gray metal door to report my findings to the nervous priest.

□ □ □ □

He was very depressed. He was an extremely neat-appearing, Asian male, twenty-six years old, and unmistakably depressed. His meticulous dress, sparsely-haired goatee, and undeniable Afro-American accent reminded me of a friend in college. However, my friend had never appeared down as he man who sat before me at Rock ledge.
The man had come to the facility because of persistent feelings of worthlessness. His thinking was organized. He knew where he was. He denied hallucinations. His old chart revealed a number of similar episodes in the past.
I looked at the small, frail man who sat quietly, dejected in the dimly lit waiting room. I felt an over-powering urge to reach out and hold him as one holds a frightened child. Instead, I asked questions.

Do you th ink you migh t h arm yourself?" I asked t he man "I don't know. "His reddened eyes were barely able to hold back his tears. I asked the question again, several times, in different ways. I needed a definite answer. A l ways the answer was the indeterminate "I don 't know." After a time, I realized that it did not matter. I had to admit him regardless. The man could not be safely sent home
The gray door opened. The small, dispirited man was led inside, silently.

CHAPTER 103

Human spirit, that wondrous entity of self-healing, overcomes the most overwhelming disease. In any sickness, it is the spirit we must treat first. For this is here that healing begins.

—the Heretic Priest, A new view of healing.

In the corridor where the staff had gathered, the mood was festive. The noise spilled over into the quiet room where I made small talk with the slight priest as the door opened

"You want to pick up on four? Somebody threatening to commit suicide." The man who had first admitted me to Rockledge spoke matter-of-factly to the priest. The man called a raucous remark into the hallway as he closed the door. Dr. Manor placed his fingers nervously in his teethas he picked up thephone.

"Hello." He said as he began chewing his nails. He listened to the receiver. "Uh-huh . . . uh-huh." The priest's eyes darted about the room anxiously, finally they came to rest on me. "I wouldn't do THA-A-T!!" Alarm caused his voice to rise in both pitch and volume.

"Here you take this." The Psychiatrist thrust the phone into my hand. I looked at him dumbfounded as he dashed from the room. What was I, a third year clinical clerk, rotating on Psychiatry, going to tell this man about to commit suicide?

I sat in the empty office, holding the receiver in mid—air. Cringing against the fear that my ears would be assaulted by the piercing report of a gunshot, I pulled the telephone to my head.

I was relieved to hear very regular breathing.

"Hello." I spoke into the receiver.

"Hello." The voice was that of a young man.

What to say now? Perhaps—~I heard you want to commit suicide. No, that would not do. Why do you want to kill yourself? No, I had to find out what brought him to this state without accepting or encouraging his suicide.

I introduced myself. "What's been going on with you?" I asked him.

"Well, I have a loaded .38 on the table in front of me and I'm going to put it to my head and pull the trigger." Sadness and sincerity saturated his voice.

I looked around the empty office, confirming for the last time that I was truly alone. "Why do you want to do that?" I spoke with more calmness than I felt.

"Nothing's going right. Everything is wrong. Nothing is right. Doc, I'm tired. I really don't want to go on like this." Sadness began to lower the volume of his voice.

"There's nothing nobody can do. I'm sorry I called. I don't know why I'm wasting your time." His voice trailed off. I could picture him hanging up the phone.

"Wait a minute!" I yelled. "Wait a minute."

"I really appreciate . . . "

"That's not what you really want to do." He paused. "If that was what you wanted to do that, you wouldn't have called here, right?"

"We—e—ell . . . "

"Look, you called here because you have a problem you want some help with."

"But . . ."
"So, let me help you."
"There's really nothing you can do."
"Then what do you have to lose by talking to me? I'm sure together we can find some solution. But I need your help. I can't do it alone. You got to help me. O.K.?"
"Well sure, we can talk."
My heart's racing eased. "What's been going on with you? You know, I don't even know your name"
"Bob."
"Bob what?"
"I'm not going to give you my last name. I don't want you to trace this call." He was right. I was trying to get information so that I could determine where he was calling. from I did not know how long he would talk. As I did not want to antagonize him, I did not press for more information. "O.K., Bob, what's been going on with you?"
"I been depressed."
"About what?"
"Everything . . . lots of things. I just moved out here. Things are kind of hard. Things ain't right between me and my old lady. She doesn't understand me. She thinks I don't care about her."
"You guys married, Bob?
"Divorced."
"How long?"
"Three years." It was not a topic on which I wanted to dwell on. Besides being a negative experience which might further lower my patient's spirits, it was too remote to alone be the major precipitant of the acute event I was witnessing. I grabbed a piece of scratch paper as I spoke. I began the task of recording minutia so that I might put together a composite identity of this man whose life hung by a slender beige telephone wire.
"Got any kids?"
"Yeah."

"How old are they?"

"Four and eight. My wife won't let me see them. She thinks I'm a bad influence on them." His tone was becoming more depressed. I jotted down the information as I asked a question.

"What kind of work do you do?"

"I'm a welder. I was just laid off from my job three weeks ago. Nobody wants to hire me." Slowly, the man who called himself Bob, but whose real name was Richard (he let it slip a few times), began to open up to a struggling student-priest. As he spoke, I wrote down one fact after another. My charge had recently been released from prison. He was divorced, unemployed, friendless, alone. He had moved to Chapel Beach (a section of Canon) within the last two months. I heard the clatter of traffic in the background. After I had talked a time, I knocked on the window frantically. The man who had let me into Rockledge appeared. I gave him a note in which I asked to have the call traced. The man returned after ten minutes. There was only one man who could trace a call in a three county area. He was two hours away. A tiring student-priest who knew he did not have two hours of conversation left with the desperate patient at the other end of the phone, looked disgustedly at the staff member then at the salmon colored walls. The door closed.

Though, I hated small talk, though I elected to remain silent rather than make idle conversation, I found anything and everything a fit topic of conversation. I talked and listened as my charge's spirits rose. I talked, talked, talked. When I knew that neither of us could talk more, I resolved to attempt to have him give up the gun.

"You don't want to harm yourself." I told him.

"No," he agreed, but I'm afraid of what I might do."

"I understand." I did not know what I should say. "I think you should get rid of the gun." I told him.

"I know, but I'm afraid to leave it in the house."

"No, Bob. I mean get it out of the house altogether." I thought for a second. "Bob do you know any of your neighbors?"

"Yeah, I know the girl who lives next door."

"Bob, I want you to do something for me."

"Yeah, what?"

"I want you give the gun to your neighbor."

"Yeah, but . . ."

"Don't worry about it. What we want to do right now is get rid of the gun the quickest and safest way possible."

"Yeah." He agreed.

"Bob, I'm going to hold onto the phone. I want you to give her the gun right now. Go ahead, I'll wait."

"O.K." I heard the phone strike a hard surface as he laid it down. There was the patter of rapid footsteps, then only the sound of an onslaught of vehicles disturbed the silence. A door closed. There was the sound of the telephone on the table again.

Bob's voice came over the phone again. "O.K., I did it."

I took my first relieved breath in two hours. "Good!" It really felt good. Suddenly, I was struck by a surge of curiosity.

"What did she say?"

"She just looked at me."

I chuckled. I spoke to my charge of seeking help, professional counseling. He adamantly refused. Still, I was glad that the life that had been held by one slender wire was on earth one more night.

As I mounted my red bicycle, emotionally drained and tired beyond measure, I felt a new contentedness. Just maybe I had fulfilled a small part of the mission of the priests of the God of Life.

The air felt fresh as the rhythmic clicking of the ball bearings of the bicycle joined the chirping of crickets and the city sounds of night.

CHAPTER 104

Too many of the battles priests fight are not with Hemorrhage, Infection, nor any of the myriad of the minions of the Priest-Foe, Death, but the useless blood-letting of Priest upon Priest

--The Heretic Priest, on Healing

the Priesthood.

It was the time of year when spring blended imperceptibly into summer, a time when the brush laden canyons of the city began to cast aside their verdant vestments in exchange for the gold of the approaching season.

A gray sun ascended in an overcast sky. My head was bowed under an enormous pessimism as I stepped across the threshold. The V.A. buzzed with the usual morning activity.

Hold your head up, I admonished myself. This is something that must be overcome. Real trouble lay ahead if I did not raise my spirits. A students who felt, as I did at that moment, that he was the victim of the combined power of the entire priest establishment, that he was going to be castigated no matter what he did, that everyone was out to get him, was headed for a difficult, if not impossible, passage. Far too often, I had seen how an attitude such as this allowed harmonious relationships with no one, not patients, staff, nor attendings. Daily arguments were followed by a decrease in the quality of work. Soon the amount of work dropped off. Rounds were missed. More rounds were missed. Finally, a dispirited student-priest stopped coming to work altogether. When he was summarily dismissed or forced to repeat the clerkship, he could see himself as nothing more than victim. He could not see how he had allowed himself to become the vehicle of his own failure.

Wait a minute, wait a minute. I paused in the doorway.

I needed somewhere to regroup, somewhere to change my attitude to a more positive one. Time was short and the V.A., despite its relative roominess, had few places where one could be alone. None of these was near at hand. I pushed open the door of a near-by restroom. I looked into the mirror. A troubled face looked back at me. Defeat and anger vied for dominance in the lines of my face.

Defeat and anger, was that all that I felt? Yes. Which was stronger? Anger? Defeat?

A thin man with gray hair and deep lines in his face beyond his age opened the door. I glared briefly at him as he sucked aggressively on a cigarette.

Anger and defeat. Anger, defeat. Anger! I would not let them defeat me before I had begun to fight. I let anger, which I had long suppressed, flow. It took over my countenance, carving lines deep and hard there. I growled. The gray-haired man looked at me oddly. Defeat would only produce defeat, but anger . . . yes, that was a fitting motion. Anger would sustain me. Anger would allow no one to tread upon me. Anger, if controlled, could bring victory where none existed. Anger allowed the dawning of arrogance. After defeat, anger, arrogance felt good. I raised my head. The door was slung open. Haughtily, I strode down the hall. I was ready for battle. It was well, I thought, that we were in a hospital.

CHAPTER 105

The priest needs unfailing stamina and an abundance of courage.

--a priest of the God of Internal

Medicine Sub-Internship.

Hunger played a disharmonious descant in my empty stomach as the noontime sun poured yellow-gold beams through tinted windows. White-uniformed figures scurried in and out of the lounge as nurses made the last-minute preparations for the pot-luck lunch. Aromas, pleasing and as varied as the international staff of 3-South, drifted across the corridor, fueling the fury in my intestines. My pen leaped forward with renewed speed

"Lunch is going to be ready in five minutes." Diane stood at the door of the sub-intern's room. I looked into a face warm and kind. I liked Diane. More than a competent nurse, she was a decent human being.

"I'll be there in a minute." She looked at me, knowing full well that my "minute" could last the better part of an hour, and smiled. I returned her smile. "I just want to finish *up* a few notes." I said, defensively. She looked dubiously at the pile of charts in front of me.

"Hurry up, it's going to get cold."

"O.K."

My work could have been left until the afternoon. Not my resident, nor anyone else would have been concerned. However, I felt uncomfortable leaving the work until later. I wished I had eaten breakfast as I did usually. My stomach bade me work faster. Forty-five minutes passed swiftly. I returned the last of the charts to the rack. Most of the food and nurses were gone. I walked into the lounge.

"Didn't think you were going to make it." Gladys looked at me through half-closed lids. An empty plate rested on her ample abdomen. "I had to finish a few charts." I answered.

"You're lucky anything is left." I looked down at several empty and near-empty bowls. "Eat." Gladys exhorted.

I needed no further invitation. I walked around the room. "What're you looking for, . . . plates?"

"Yes."

"Here." Under her used plate was a clean one. I took the proffered dish. I used a large spoon to dig into a bowl of seasoned rice.

Diane appeared in the doorway. "You have an admission." She looked at me.

"What is it?" I asked

"Is he stable?" Stable in this case denoted that he was not acutely ill and could wait a few minutes. "Yeah."

"O.K., I'll be there in a minute."

"O.K." Diane left. Lung cancer that dread disease ubiquitous to the Veterans Administration hospitals usually required nothing in the way of emergent treatment. If Diane said he was stable, I was sure he was. Still, I felt guilty. I had not laid eyes on the patient. I would have been faulted by none except my own conscience had I waited until after I had eaten to see him. The spoon filled with rich brown rice and well-cooked meat, was suspended above my plate. I swore under my breath. I returned the spoon to the bowl, then placed my empty plate on the table.

"Oh, go ahead and eat!" Gladys called to me.

"I'll get something later." The history and physical took only half an hour. I was pleased with myself. I was getting better. Mr. Kenny's history varied little from that of so many other men I had worked up with his disease. He was about fifty and had smoked since he had been a teenager. By the time he had his first symptom, he already had wide-spread, inoperable disease. He enjoyed the attention of his first grandchild, a bright-eyed little girl who shared a special love with her grandfather. He had worked hard all his life and was in the V.A. to receive treatment almost as unhealthy as his disease. My charge was a likable, frightened, small man who had never before been in a hospital. I spent a few extra minutes talking with him, trying to allay some of his fears. The cancer doctors would be by to see him later in the day.

I wrote a few routine admitting orders, then returned to the lounge. While I reviewed his old chart and wrote his history and physical, I could eat lunch. My watering mouth hung open at the sight that awaited me. Except for a single cold egg roll, all the food was gone. I stood in the empty room in disbelief for several seconds. With an egg roll in one hand and my patient's old chart in the other, I retired to the sub-intern's room. Slowly the sheets of paper were filled with the ink of my pen.

"You better come!" Diane stood in the doorway. From her tone and expression, I knew there was serious trouble. "It's Mr. Kenny." She told me as we walked briskly. There was a flurry of activity at the patient's door.

"He's really coughing up blood."

The man, who was ashen and becoming cyanotic, was indeed coughing up blood, at least an ounce at a time. Diane bent over the man's arm. "I'm trying to get a line." She told me.

"Good." My heart galloped within my chest. "We need a second line in the other arm. Also, a type and cross, and CBC."

"I'll do that." Someone called out.

"We need a stat blood gas, EKG, some 0 2." I ordered, almost by reflex, as I listened to the man's chest.

"How're you doing.?" I yelled to the patient.

"O.K., doctor." He called to me. His face was a frank blue.

"O.K., Mr. Kenny." The situation was beyond me. Tony Barrett, my resident was in clinic.

I returned to the sub-intern's room, leaving the phone clear at the nurse's station for the emergency.

"I need to talk to Tony Barrett." I spoke into the phone.

"Is it important?" The perturbed voice at the other end asked.

"YES, it's important!" I yelled. "I need to talk with him right away about one of his patients!"

"One moment. I'll get him."

Long seconds passed. "Hello?" It was Tony.

"I think you better come up. This guy I just admitted doesn't look good."

"The guy with lung CA?"

"Yeah."

"He's coughed up half a unit of blood in the last five minutes."

Footsteps were running down the hall. As Diane passed my room, she yelled two words. "He's coding!" My heart was out of control.

"What's going on?!" The resident demanded.

"Tony, he just . . . " My voice rose an octave. "CODED!"I heard the resident swear just before both phones went click. Feet from all directions ran toward the patient's room as the announcement went out over the loud speaker. I arrived just in time to see my patient empty his mouth of more than a pint of blood. His head went flat against the bed. He was deep, deep blue. He was not breathing.

"Bag him!" a resident who was the first member of the code team to arrive called out. A large black bag with a tight-fitting mask was placed over the patient's face.

She felt his neck. "No pulse. You want to pump, please?" She spoke to an intern who promptly began a rhythmic pushing on the man's chest.

The two bedded room was fast becoming packed. "Anyone who is not a member of the code team, please leave!" The resident called out. Reluctantly, a few people left. She repeated her order louder. I was not a member of the code team and could probably do little, if anything, but I was not going to desert my charge in the middle of a code. She continued giving orders as I watched.

"Does anyone here know this patient?" She called out.

"I know the patient." I swallowed audibly. She gave me a measuring look. "What is his history?" My voice cracked several times as I spoke. "He is a fifty-three year old man with non-resectable lung cancer, metastatic to the hilum and both lungs. He may have other mets as well . . . He's here for work-up now."

She thought of the information I had given her. "Are you sure you want to resuscitate this man?" She looked me full in the face.

The question was a profound one. If the man did not die there on that bed at that moment, he would die shortly after no one knew how much suffering. Would we be doing anything more than simply prolonging the agony of a protracted death?

It was a question as deep as the holy mission of the priesthood. It was a question I was not prepared to grapple with as the priest stood at the bedside fighting toe-to-toe with Death.

"Ye-es." I stammered. I was not willing to take the responsibility for my charge's life. She looked at me with an expression filled with sympathy and knowing. The breathless figure of Tony Barrett, my resident, was thrust into the doorway. "How's he doing." The resident asked. The man had not responded to any of our efforts. The priest in charge of the code team told Tony this. The efforts of the priests continued a few minutes more. There was not a flicker of life in the man.

"That's enough." Tony tapped the intern who straddled the man's chest. "You can stop now." The intern turned to look at the resident, the other priests in the room.

"That's it." The priest who headed the code team called out.

"Thank you, everybody." Tony called. The priests left the room one by one. Each sought a basin. Each tried, through vigorous scrubbing, to remove the tainted touch of Death.

I looked upon my charge, now still in the arms of the great priest adversary. I wanted neither to stay nor to leave. Tony stood next to me. "There was nothing anybody could do." He said quietly, then left.

It was true, I knew. Mr. Kenny had had no chance. Death had laid a perfect ambush and had deftly taken my charge.

At least, I had not delayed in seeing him. I would not have to bear that burden of guilt. Still, as I turned to leave the room, peace was far away.

CHAPTER 106

The inherent qualities of Divinity do not determine God's form. It is the willingness of each individual to accept Divinity which determines which forms God will take.

—the Heretic Priest, On the nature of Deity

My **second passage** through the halls of the God of Internal Medicine was not like the first. I had expected the worst. Each day I expected a scathing castigation for no crimes in particular. Instead, each morning I met a face, sleepy like my own, which belonged to one then a second resident. Both residents were interested in caring for our patient and seeing that the two sub-interns got a good education. Cases were carefully selected for us for their maximal teaching potential. Tony Barrett was only present for a week. His successor, Jim Lindsey, was a Vietnam Veteran who spoke with a pronounced Texas accent. Jim had an uncanny talent for cutting through the trappings directly to the meat of the issue. We had many lively discussions on anything from politics to war to medicine. The resident-priest ran rounds briskly. As we were given the responsibilities of interns, Jim expected us to act as interns. We were expected to know every detail about each of our patients every day. Jim accepted no less than our best and, in turn, gave nothing but his. I liked Jim immensely for many reasons--his forthright honesty, his fairness, his patience. I liked him because he allowed the two student-priests under him to grow. I liked Jim because he was the first priest who treated me as a priest. The differences between my first and second passages went further than the residents. The conferences which I was required to attend (the same as those of the interns) had an altogether different character. It was as if having passed through the baptismal fires of the third year, I was now considered a member of the inner club. The weekly meetings with the department chief (the third-year equivalent to Ground Rounds) was cast in an altogether different light. When we arrived, we were greeted with wedges from the best delicatessen in the area rather than pre-lunch grumbling stomachs. The first question was not what did the urinalysis show, but rather, was the food to our liking? If not, or if we were tired of this fare, the food would be ordered from another vendor. The major item of business was not the discomfiture of the presenting student-priest, but the teaching of the newest members of the Department. There was evident in these meetings an esprit de corps that I had never seen among the priests of Internal Medicine. I began to see in others an excitement in the problems of internal medicine which I had experience only alone before. Each week I looked forward to these conferences. I considered a career in internal medicine.

Though I was already determined to do well no matter what the obstacles, I was driven even farther by the positive attitudes of those about me. Each night, my fellow sub-intern and I worked until eight or nine at night, sometimes ten or eleven. I was often so tired that my bones ached, but I loved every minute of it. The more I worked, the more I learned and the more I realized I already knew.

More than knowledge, I received something I had not known from the priests of the God of Internal Medicine--praise. Both my resident and my attending commended my work.

□ □ □ □

It was near the end of my rotation on Medicine. I had just presented a case during rounds. As I walked away to complete my ward work, I heard my name called. The attending priest, newly-arrived from the premiere training hospital in the country, beckoned me toward him. Quickly on the defensive, my mind searched for something I had done wrong or had neglected to do. I steeled myself for the coming criticism. "Yes?" I stood stoically before the attending-priest. "You're going to be applying for programs soon, right?"

"Yes."

"Well, I just wanted to let you know that I think you've done a splendid job. When you need a letter of recommendation, let me know. I'll be glad to write one for you."

I was dumbfounded. I managed to stammer, "Thank you!" I shook his hand earnestly. He smiled, before turning toward his office.

"ALRIGHTI!!!" It was all I could do not to race down the hall slapping the hand of every passer-by. That he would have consented to write a letter for me after I had groveled, as tradition demanded, would have been good fortune. This total break with protocol, he approaching me was more than I had ever expected. "ALRIGHTI" I repeated. I smiled broadly as I walked back to the wards. I was three feet off the ground.

CHAPTER 107

I have a habit of surviving under the most adverse conditions. Sometimes it surprises even me.

--a student-priest of the Semi-Secret Society

Summer the season of my birth, the season I loved above all others, the season when the spring seedlings thrive and grow, summer, the season filled with seemingly endless days and eternal, rose colored sunsets, summer the season filled with living, was also filled with work. I began my second sub-internship, this one in the Medical Intensive Care Unit (MICU) a scant week after finishing my first sub-internship on the medical wards. It was July and that meant a new academic year, new house staff, and much confusion.

Lance Schultz, a tall, thin priest with sharp, angular Germanic features was the resident in charge of the MICU. It was ironic that Lance should be my resident as two weeks before he had been one of two interns to present a case at the weekly Cardiology conference. I had been the second "intern". With the start of the new academic year, Lance had progressed to medical resident, I to the fourth year.

There was a joke that was very popular among house staff. Jim Lindsey had been the first to tell it to me. "How are thc ICU resident and James Bond alike?" He had asked. I did not know. "They both have a license to kill."

Lance evidently took the admonition implied in this joke quite seriously. The trepidation of the priest coupled with the desire of the two full-fledged interns to learn procedures, allowed me with little to do except attend the myriad of daily rounds. In fact, it was only after three weeks of gentle and not so gentle arm-twisting on my part and a direct order from the attending that I was allowed to do anything more than a cursory history and physical.

Though he was a major road block to my hands-on experience with patients, he had one outstanding characteristic--he talked. He talked to me about anything and everything that went on in the MICU. No question was too unimportant or too complicated. I was a dry sponge thirsty for knowledge. Knowledge flowed freely from the priest. I pestered him with questions virtually every minute of every day, and I learned. Every third night we were on-call together. We would talk about medicine until four A.M. Each morning when sleep and tiredness finally overcame us both.

One of the two interns was Jane Forrest, a slender, blond mother of two who had put a husband through law school before going to medical school. She had been ranked number one in my entering class. She knew what had befallen me in Pathology. She knew that I was yet a fourth-year student while she was an intern, a full-fledged priest. I was awed by the marked difference in our stations, in a system almost as rigid in its adherence to rank as the military. Initially, I experienced a great deal of discomfort in her presence. I deferred to her often, while she, either unaware of my discomfort or ignoring it, treated me fully as an equal. For this I was grateful. To my surprise and delight, a camaraderie soon developed between us.

□ □ □ □

The day was golden and delicious. I kept fighting the urge to slow down and enjoy more of the gentle greenness of the Academy's almost rural setting. A quick glance at my watch pushed the notion quickly from my head. I decided to have lunch and look in on a few people at the main campus of the medical school before returning to the University Hospital and the MICU. I had stopped briefly at the office of the Minority Recruitment Program to say hello to its director, Martha Livingston, and her secretary Mabel Furst. I stood in the doorway, refusing to sit down, as I knew it was altogether too easy for Martha and I to get into a three-hour conversation. I called good-bye after only a few minutes. There was no line at the cafeteria. As I looked for a place to sit, I saw him at a table alone. We both smiled as I approached.

"Hey, what's happening, man?" I called out.

"What's going on?" I took a seat next to Tim. I could see that despite his gladness to see me, he was sad. In the ensuing months after Medicine 1, I felt a growing kinship with Tim and Louis. Louis and Tim had been close before, but I felt that the shared clerkship had brought them closer as well. I was very glad for the good feelings our times together had engendered. Tim and I made small talk for a few minutes between mouthfuls.

"You seem a little down, man. What's bothering you?" I asked. "Nothing . . . just lots of problems." Something was bothering him. I could pull it out with a little effort, I knew.

"Hi!" I followed the arm attached to the descending plate. A face I only vaguely recognized, one belonging to a fourth-year medical student, smiled at Tim and me broadly.

"Hi."

"Hi." The student pulled a chair to the table. "I'm only going to stay a minute." He said before stuffing the first piece of a tuna sandwich into his mouth. Tim smiled pleasantly. I looked at my watch. I had already stretched my conference and lunch break to a maximum. The van to the U. was leaving in ten minutes. I said little as Tim and the other student talked.

A few minutes passed. "Well, I've got to go." I said. I wanted to stay.

"Take it easy." Tim told me.

"You, too, man." I returned.

Walking briskly back to the waiting van, I made a mental note to call Tim soon. As the small bus got underway, my thoughts swiftly turned to the MICU and the beauty of the turquoise sky.

THE THIRD YEAR

CHAPTER 108

Self versus non-self. If we were once able to find how the body distinguishes between the two, we would have the answer to a multitude of diseases related to the immune system.

--academy lectures, Immunity and Disease

Thirty-seven year old Black male with two year history of high blood pressure . . . No, no, that was not right. Thirty-seven year old hypertensive male on a kidney machine because . . . no. Thirty-seven year old, all too healthy-appearing male who by the grace of God should not be here. These were my thoughts as I looked down upon Willie's body. He was being transferred from the Surgical Intensive Care Unit to the Medical Intensive Care Unit. This was not a good sign as the surgeons often passed their long term chronic and non-viable patients onto Medicine. Willie was my patient for the second time in my career. In the MICU we poured drugs into Willie to counteract the fight his body put up against the foreign tissue in his pelvis, tissue which kept him alive. Willie's body was rejecting his transplanted kidney.

I spoke briefly with Willie. After an initial hello and how are you doing?, I had ended the conversation, sensing my charge's tiredness.

Something bothered me about Willie. It was more than the resentment and humiliation of a man with only a wash cloth over his genitals so that access to the multiplicity of tube and wires would not be hampered. It was not that his kidneys had been decimated in two years by hypertension. It was not the dull, spiritless eyes I knew to be full of life on his good days. It was not the twenty-two devastating medical problems. It was not the look that begged please go away whenever anyone approached. It was more than these that gripped my stomach whenever I saw him, that made me maintain a distance from him.

It was not until the third day that he was in the MICU when he asked for and received yet another tube when he could not breathe on his own that I came to realize what it was that made me uneasy about him.

"Poor guy!" I spoke to Rachel, the head nurse. "Look at this!" I ran my hand down both sides of the paper which told of his illnesses.

"I know." She moaned. "And so young!"

I looked again at Willie. Though I knew his age, I did not realize until that moment how young he was. Looking at Willie closely, I realized that he appeared much younger than thirty-seven. He looked as someone twenty-five--my own age.

I, like Willie, was Black and male. Further I had A higher risk of developing hypertension as I had a family member who had the disease. As I looked at Willie, I wondered was I looking into my own future?

Uneasiness was a barrier I could neither penetrate nor dispel.

CHAPTER 109

Grant us, your priests, wisdom, courage, and strength as we guide our charges through the domain of disease.

--a prayer of the priests of Life

Lines of tiredness were etched deeply into Louis' face. He was the Cardiac Care Unit sub-intern. When he was on-call he covered the MICU as well. He met me in the hall as I made my way to the MICU before morning work rounds. Weariness was in his voice.

"Willie died last night."

Shock, dismay sent my thoughts tumbling. Any denial was precluded by the emotionless, matter-of-fact-ness of the student-priest's voice. "What . . . what happened?"

"He, coded last night."

I tried to swallow. "Yeah?"

"He coded THREE TIMES!" He shook three fingers before my face for emphasis. Disgust and anger were in Louis' voice. "They worked on him for three hours. The last time they didn't bring him back." Louis looked at the floor, shook his head. "I was glad he died." There was no malevolence in his voice.

I was taken back by Louis' statement. My concern with his statement was more personal than my concern for my patient. How dare he be glad my patient was dead? "What do you mean?" I asked.

"George, he had suffered too damn much. It was time for them to let him die." I felt a little ashamed for having considered my own vanity and not my patient first. I fought agreement with Larry's words, but I knew that he was right. Willie had been on an inexorably downhill course for some time. I also knew that no life worth saving could possibly have survived three cardiac arrests in a single night.

Louis looked over the walls vaguely. His eyes seemed to have lost the ability to focus after the strain of the night's work.

"When did he die?" I asked.

"About three-thirty. He was already dead before that."

"You look tired."

"Yeah, we didn't get any sleep last night." A few seconds passed. "I'm going to get me some breakfast before rounds." I smiled, remembering the large meals Louis could eat and not put on a single pound.

"Yeah, you look like you could use some and some rest, too."

Louis swore softly. "I'm not going to get any rest until tonight sometime. We got company coming this evening." Louis half dragged his feet over the gray tiles as he ambled down the hallway. "Take it easy." He called.

"You, too."

Immaculately white sheets covered the haunting empty bed. The clipboard was bare. Only the tell-tale red eyes of two nurses evinced the passing of one of the bravest men I have ever known. The women's eyes were no small tribute as MICU nurses, living daily with the rapaciousness of Death, did not often shed tears.

Woody, the spirited warrior with an unquenched zeal for life, had touched us all.

CHAPTER 110

We who serve the God of Life must end the days of Healing. We must move beyond repairing that which is diseased. We must seek the highest level of the God-Self within .

--the Heretic Priest, The priesthood's mission

The morning was a hazy yellow. I drove my small light-colored station wagon to the oceanside neighborhood where Grace worked. I was in the middle of a morning full of errands for which I had been granted time off.

Slivers of pale sun shimmered lazily over waves which rose and fell as if savoring the fleeting edge of a pleasant slumber. Had my mind not been fixed to the clock, it would have been a good morning for peaceful meditation and quiet reflective walks along the shore. I sped past the inlet to Church Bay with barely a second glance at the bright and colorful sail boats gliding within the channel.

The growling of my car's small engine came to a halt in front of a dress shop. Ann was waiting outside. As I walked toward her, she lifted a face filled with tears. I rushed to put my arms around her.

"Sweetheart, what's the matter?"

"Did . . . Louis . . . get . . . you?" she asked between sobs.

"No."

The sobs continued. "Tim . . . is . . . dead!"

"What?!" Who Tim? Not *our* Tim.

Grace bawled unrestrained as I held her. Her tears, the racking of her body were an immutable verification of my worst fears. No, not Tim. But, yes, it was Tim. I needed to know more.

"What happened, Gracie?"

"He . . . committed . . . suicide." I questioned her no further. She was incapable of saying more.

During the next few days, I was able to gather the details of Tim's death. He had been found by the Highway Patrol who had been alerted when he had not returned home after several days. He had been found in his automobile in Discovery, a town eight-hundred miles from Canon, famous for its deep green forests which rolled into the sea and gold mines. The student-priest had ended his life by diverting his vehicle's exhaust into the passenger compartment.

Tim had left a tape recording. My fear of its message pervaded even my shock at Tim's passing. As I was the only person I blamed more than the priests of Internal Medicine for my friend's death, I imagined an unflinching, finger pointing directly at me. I thought of the strange circumstances which had brought Tim's life and mine together. The odds were very much against our meeting as we did. To the great embarrassment of all sides, the internecine politics of the priest academy had resulted in only one student of African descent out of one hundred in the class which entered the year before my arrival in Canon. The student had left after a few months. His departure left not only a mark against Canon which took years to erase, but also a void at the level of student participation, an integral part of the admissions process.

I had been in the Minority Recruitment Office the day Tim had come for his interview and was asked to give him a tour of the campus. I had been impressed with his great height and his quiet gentleness. I had shown the best side of the school as only an insider could. I had not been surprised later to learn that Tim had chosen Canon. There were very few students whom I spoke to as I had Tim and who were accepted who did not choose Canon.

Because I had been instrumental in Tim's coming to Canon, I felt a special obligation to watch out for him. Now, he was eight-hundred miles away, cold and dead.

I had failed.

□ □ □ □

Grace was going. She was adamant. She was going to Tim's funeral. Though I knew she loved Tim as much as I, I was surprised. Louis was planning to go, as well. He outlined the route we would have to take to arrive in the small town with no major airport and only twice weekly scheduled flights. The trip would require a two day lay over. I listened, wordlessly, to the plans of both Grace and Louis, knowing that I did not have the money, nor the means of obtaining it, for a trip half the distance.

An unsettled night called forth a crimson dawn. As there were no relatives in Discovery, no one to make arrangements, Tim's family yielded to practicality. He was to be buried in Calmante, a town where family did exist. I had never before heard of the town, but it was within a day's drive. Grace wanted to go. I did not, but did not tell her so. I had had enough of dead people. One could never bring them back. Still, I knew Grace wanted to go. We were going.

CHAPTER 111

Before their rift, the priests of the God of Life and the priests of the God of the After-Life were one. However, a dichotomy arose within the priesthood. The priests of Life absolved themselves from human spirit, claiming physiology, chemistry, and biochemistry as their realm. They forgot that the physical form was only an expression of the Divine one. The priests of the After-Life felt that the only life which mattered was that lived after our death in this one. They too had their blindness, for they forsook today, forgetting that Divinity expresses itself in each of us every moment of every day.

--writings of the Priest who
served both Life and Beyond

It was the first time I had seen the priest since he had been guest speaker in a second-year elective. The protestant minister, a priest of the God of the After-Life, measured his audience through gaunt brown eyes. The florescent lights flickered briefly off the thick black-rimmed glasses as a restive quiet descended. The conference room overflowed with the priests, student-priests, nurses, staff of every specialty, every God which served in the House of the God of Life. The priest of the God of After-Life, cleared his throat. He watched as the quiet rose in volume until even the hushed whispers could be heard. He passed his face slowly over the room once again. A deafening silence hung in the air.

I looked up from the yellow, waxed linoleum floor. My eyes rose slowly encountering the priest's black shirt, the spot of white at his neck, the red line of his thin lips. The priest waited, appraising his audience through thick distorted lenses. His eyes flickered over mine, briefly.

When the silence could contain itself no more, when it threatened to engulf the priest and those who sat before him, when the combined weight of anticipation of those in the room could be held in check no longer, the priest spoke. He began by saying how dear Tim had been to those gathered. He spoke of the tragic circumstances of the student-priest's demise. He acknowledged, without conviction, the burden of sadness we all shared. He spoke briefly, vaguely of Tim the person. I realized, as the priest spoke, that he had not known Tim. I realized that he was but an impromptu actor with no lines and little preparation enlisted by the priests of the God of Life to aid them in absolving themselves of blame. I was deeply angered that this priest of the God of the After-Life could perpetrate so shallow a sham.

The priest continued. I lifted my eyes from the dull polished floor. With an expression which was both stern and unyielding, the priest looked directly into my face. He admonished ". . . and let us not act out of anger." I met the priest's gaze with smoldering eyes. The priest looked away. The service ended a short time after.

I looked about me. The uniforms were a myriad of colors denoting every station from housekeeping to priest. I was struck by how the love of my comrade cut so clearly across the rigid lines of rank and class.

Those who served the God of Life shuffled out slowly. A few offered conversation. I took my leave, preferring the solace of my own company.

CHAPTER 112

Priests are simply human, filled with the frailty and divinity that that term implies.
--a priest of the God of Life.

Time ground slowly, gnawing at my intestines. What could I do? Tim was dead. I could not bring him back. Yet if I said, did nothing, my silence would be an affirmation to the blamelessness of the priests of Medicine 1. But what could I do that was not an empty protest nor a feeble attempt to absolve my own guilt?

I had changed during my stay at the Academy of the Priests of Life. Two years before, I had been an active participant in the inner workings of the school, an agent for change for the better. I remembered a sober-faced meeting with one of the deans who had blocked every effort of a coalition of faculty and students to reverse the decimation of the ranks of students of color over a three-year period. I had arrived without an appointment. He had invited me into his office for what I knew was a face-down. The seasoned, political in-fighter was pitted against the unfledged, would-be priest. Alone, armed with nothing more than the conviction that the dean was wrong, that his motives were among the basest to which humans succumbed and that I was doing as my conscience bade me, I had faced down the gray-haired dean. While doing this I had not considered the possible consequences. I had acted because I felt that I was right. Looking back, I knew my actions had been brave, as well. How long had it been since I had felt such a surge of pride or courage?

My thoughts went back to Medicine 1, my deal with the priests. Though in the end I had not been penalized academically, the bargain had skillfully skirted the central issue--the treatment of Louis, Tim and I. Was I bought off by the promise of an easier time ahead as a medical sub-intern or had I simply accepted a good offer? Was time making me wise or complacent? No answer came. The silence was unsettling.

What seemed like many days, but which was no more than two or three, passed. I always got as far as the first few lines then confusion would overwhelm me.

"Dear Dr. Solomon, "The purpose of this letter is to inform you of some of the circumstances surrounding the death of Timothy Birdsong. . .

"It is not, nor can it be the role of a school of medicine to remedy all wrongs, social or personal, one of its trainees might encounter on the road to being a physician. Nor can the school, in the brief period of four years, equip an individual with the tools by which to withstand the onslaught of those wrongs. This responsibility must be borne by parents as they rear the individual, by other family members, loved ones, friends and most importantly by the individual himself . . . "

No, that was not the approach I wanted.

"Dear Dr. Solomon,

"It cannot be tolerated that an institution which claims as its purpose the training of practitioners of the most noble of calling, stand itself the cause of monumental suffering of humans under its sway. Unfortunately, this is precisely the position of the School of Medicine in the life of one Timothy Birdsong . . . " No, that was not quite what I wanted, either.

The only thing I could definitely decide was that the letter would be addressed to the Dean of the School of Medicine, the highest of the high priests of the academy.

□ □ □ □

"Did Helen find you?" Ruth asked as I arrived at the Cardiology office.

"No." I fingered the unfinished letter in my pocket.

"She was just here a second ago. I thought maybe you passed her in the hall."

"No." I took off my white coat and hooked it behind the straight-backed chair. Ruth looked as if she wanted to talk.

"Do you know what it was she wanted?" I asked.

"Yes." She held the book she had been reading when I walked in to her chest. She put the book down and pulled her chair closer to mine. I turned to face her. The student-priest spoke. "I don't know how you felt, but a lot of people really felt cheated after the service for Tim." I looked deep into the woman's face. "A group of us want a meeting where we can all express our feelings about what happened. We thought you would want to be involved." Ruth looked earnestly in my face. A light, soft, pain-laden, vulnerable, was in her blue eyes. I was surprised by the warmth of my colleague. Also, I was taken back again by the wide-spread popularity of my colleague. Somehow, I had expected only we of African descent to mourn his passing.

"Yes, I would like that very much. Thanks." I smiled. "Is there anything you would like me to do?"

"No." She smiled. "It's all been arranged."

CHAPTER 113

One of the major justifications for the existence of priesthoods is their humanizing effect upon governance.
--the Heretic Priest

It was seven o'clock. I had timed my arrival to coincide with the beginning of the meeting. Thirty to forty people were gathered in the student lounge of the main campus of the priest academy.

The room's dull green carpet had a relaxing restfulness about it. I had spent many hours in the room during breaks and late at night after classes. Sometimes as the clock pushed far beyond midnight, I had sat alone in the large room translating single-stringed guitar melodies onto the warn keyboard of the mahogany piano. Often passers-by would come and go unaware that I sat motionless in the shadows. There was an intimacy of the room which went beyond my years of familiarity with it, which was more than the pleasant meals and the pleasant times with friends which I had enjoyed there. There was more than these in my good feelings about the room. The room, though an integral part of the building that housed most of the basic science research as well as the medical school administration, had somehow managed to be separate and distinct from these. Somehow, despite monumental pressures to encroach upon its space, the room had remained whole and had maintained an identity all its own. I liked the room. Conversation was light and amicable. On the near edge of the room's upper deck sat Garret Frank. Recessed lamps set in the ceiling left alternate patches of yellow-white light and semi-darkness. I smiled as I approached the priest-confessor. I moved to a place a little off from him in a hidden corner. Several faces caught my eye as I moved toward my seat. Frank Solomon, the Dean of the School of Medicine was present. So too, were the deans of admissions and academic affairs. The newly announced future dean of student affairs whom I remembered most for his razor wit as he had chaired the admissions committee was also at the gathering. The chief of service at the V.A., the man who was second only to Lovela Ground in the hierarchy of the priests of Internal Medicine, sat in a far corner of the room. Beside him sat Stand, one of the few priests of his house who had shown us any kindness.

I sat in an unlit corner, watching. One of the deans spoke. His tone was soft, subdued, searching. He said that he was amenable to any format for the meeting. Frank Solomon, the highest of the high priests, spoke briefly. He wanted to know why such a tragedy had occurred, what might be done to prevent another in the future? He ended by stating that his door was always open. There was a simple earnestness in the man which could not be denied.

It was time for the students to speak. Most had never before been face to face with the Dean. Most were awed by the presence of the man who wielded more power than any other human in their lives and the lives of those about them.

Unlike most of my colleagues, I had spoken with the Dean on a few occasions. I had found him to be honest, forthright, fair. I had found him to be a man bound by his word. My dealing with him had been a refreshing reaffirmation of the better qualities of the priesthood and humanity. It was as much because of these qualities of the man as his position as Dean that I had addressed my unfinished letter to him.

Silence hung awkwardly in the air until Helen spoke. Her words, thick and clumsy initially, flowed smoothly as she struck upon the desired timbre of her message. She spoke of the students feeling of being cheated at the memorial service. She mentioned in only the vaguest terms the unpleasant experiences Tim had suffered at the academy. Other students echoed her words and asked what was being done to prevent further suicides? Another student-priest who had taken his life the previous year was mentioned. Faculty members interjected comments and made sincere offers of aid to any student who felt that they had emotional problems.

Sporadically, Helen cast nervous glances into the shadows where I sat. I listened silently as discussion wandered from the factors which had led my friend to commit suicide to self-congratulations on the support systems at the academy.

I wondered if I should speak. Would not my tongue fail me as it had in my unfinished letter to Solomon?

A number of comments were made regarding Tim's personal problems, his homosexuality. The V.A. chief of service smiled contentedly in his distant corner. Conversation lapsed into silence.

No one had mentioned Medicine 1.

"I have a few things to say." Necks twisted, peering into the semi-darkness in which I sat. I moved forward into the glare of the yellow-white beam. I was surprised by the strength and clarity of my voice. "I think that there are some things that happened to Tim that really need to be addressed directly. Tim's death didn't just happen. It was the result of what was for Tim an insurmountable amount of anguish which in large part was due to events which took place at this medical school, particularly in Medicine 1.

"Having spent no small amount of time with him on that clerkship, I know some of the things he went through. Daily he got it from the attending on down about how poor a student he was, that he had no hopes of becoming an even mediocre physician. Daily, the doctors of our team and those in the Department of Medicine would go out of their way to say particularly derogatory things about him.

"This is nowhere better exemplified than on his written evaluations. They were nothing more than a slanderous, baseless attack on Tim as an individual. They do not read like evaluations, but rather they testify to the base, small-minded attitudes of those who wrote them.

"One has to ask oneself if these documents could pertain to any student who went through two years of rigorous basic science training at Canon? No, these are nothing more than personal insults against one Timothy Birdsong.

"It would be unjust of me to lay the entire burden of guilt at the door of the School of Medicine. However, speaking as one who spoke with Tim, spent time with Tim and shared those experiences with him, I would not be true to him or myself if I did not state unequivocally that a major portion of the blame for Tim's death arose directly from events that transpired in Medicine 1." The silence was profound, awe-inspiring. I looked around the room at everyone and no one. Anger blinded me to faces and welled as thick as rain in my eyes. If anything else was said, I did not hear it. I stayed until the priests and student-priests rose, signaling the end of the meeting. I sped to the door.

I vowed to die rather than shed a tear that any of those gathered could see. Though anger boiled within me threatening to overflow the bounds of my burning eyes, I kept my promise.

A yellow Dodge cut ribbons in the night with eyes of white fire. I was angry at one person more than the priests who had mentally brutalized my comrade. I was angry at me.

CHAPTER 114

Their championing of the rights of those with neither power nor voice, their support of unpopular causes, predicated solely upon their concern for the well-being of their charges is a considerable source of pressure and power outside the lines of governing structures which can greatly alleviate suffering. This power of priests goes beyond the dichotomy of the priests of Life and After-Life. It has no regard for deity, sect, nationality. It is universal.

However, with this power comes responsibility. We must use this power consistently and conscientiously for the betterment of our charges or lose it altogether.

--the Heretic Priest, Responsibility and power

The yellow sun rose in a sky clear except for the figures of sparrows foraging for food. The usual early haze was already burned off though the morning was only half gone.

I listened to the sporadic coughing of the yellow station wagon. To either side of the gray highway lay great expanses of low, rolling, dirt-brown hills stripped of the gold green vestments of early summer.

The car went above sixty-five again. I winced. I looked at Gracie. She drove with intensity. I listened to the sounds of the car. Some three years before, I had nick-named it the "hungry tiger" because of the humming-growl of its engine. However, as we drove to Calmante, the sound of the vehicle was a prolonged mechanical wheeze. I closed my eyes to block out the approaching reality of both Tim's funeral and the break of our car. I patted my back pocket, comforted by the knowledge that I had enough money there for bus fare back to Canon.

□ □ □ □

White block letters on a green sign indicated Calmante, the town we had driven five hours to find. The air was hot and still. The passing of endless cars on the worn highway stirred the air only for fleeting seconds. Our yellow car pulled into a service station. A young man, his face red from countless unshaded hours in the sun, looked up from the back end of a pick-up truck. He held a rusted silver nozzle to a hole in the vehicle's side. I rolled down the dirty window of my car. I asked where might we find the cemetery we sought? He held up a long finger as he indicated that the cemetery was not far. He continued to pump gas. I thanked him.

We arrived at the cemetery only minutes before the appointed time. We looked over flat grounds cluttered with gray, granite stones. There were a few single people, but no gathering.

We inquired in the office. The service had been postponed we were told, the location changed. We started once again. We moved slowly to the funeral home where Tim's body lay.

The building, largely hidden by shrubs, was on the corner of a quiet residential neighborhood. We parked in the shade avoiding the oppressive heat as much as we could. The funeral parlor did not smell like a house of Death. Perhaps my long association with the dying had dulled my senses to the odor. As I opened the door uncertainly, I saw what could easily have been the inside of a wedding chapel. "Hello-o-o!" a thin woman with whispers of gray in her brown hair greeted us nervously.

Grace became an unmoving statue once inside the door. I spoke to the woman. "We are here to see the body of Tim Birdsong."

The woman hesitated.

"This way," she said finally, indicating a carpeted walkway between rows of white pews. We approached the front of the draped room. The casket seemed small, much too small for the man whom had seemed, in life, a giant. We neared the end of the walkway, peering into the coffin as if we were looking over the edge of a great precipice. Finally, Tim lay before us.

His body, thinner than I had ever seen it, was arrayed in a flowing white robe and pants. He could have graced the throne of a great and proud nation had he been born in another time, another continent. Instead, in the blossoming of his youth, he lay in a sleep from which he would never awaken.

Tim, get up from there, I thought. Get out of that coffin! Tim, quit playing around. I fully expected him to sit up and say, as he had on so many occasions, "I fo-o-oled you, didn't I?!" I must have waited for half of a minute for Tim to sit up, call to me. There was only a disheartening silence. Tim lay still, not moving.

Grace sobbed softly. I felt overwhelmed by sadness and anger. We turned to leave. As I reached the end of the walkway, I turned once again, half-expectantly. The silent stillness was interrupted only by Grace's stifled cries as I held her.

As I opened the door, the heat of Calmante fell heavily upon us once more.

CHAPTER 115

With a child's passing, a bit of hope dies as well.

--an unnamed poet

The funeral home was hushed. A small woman with dark brown skin, Tim's sister, spoke. Her demeanor was strained and business-like. The burden of grief showed in the nearly smooth lines of the placid facade she presented to those who watched. As requested by Tim, she told us, there would not be funeral services as such. However, the tall man whom I had called friend, wanted to share his last words, in the form of a tape, with those who had gathered. She sat down quietly before the glistening white casket as music drifted over the room. The song, then popular and often heard on the radio, began with a soft collage of notes from a keyboard. The voice of Billy Joel lifted into the air. He sang "Just the Way You Are". The melodic sounds continued for a few minutes. As the last note died away, Tim's voice was heard. My eyes went from the back of Tim's sister's head to the coffin whose contents were hidden by a cascade of flowers.

He was sad, he said. His voice broke for the first of several times, sobs filled the tape. His tears were shared by the moistened eyes of many in the room. He mentioned several friends by name. He spoke of his roommate. Carl, "You were the best friend a man could ever have . . ." He spoke of many other people. I recognized only a few. Each was given a few kind words. Notably missing were the names of anyone from the school of priests except a hulking surgeon with skillful hands. I did not know that the priest had become Tim's adviser and friend. Tim thanked the priest for trying to help him and apologized for being unable to keep the promises he had made. There was an expression of gratitude to Joanna. It was not until some months later that I recognized the name as that which belonged to a woman who worked in the office of a priest of the Joined Hands and who, with her employer, had befriended and aided many student-priests.

Many, many times Tim expressed his love for family and friends. He asked that no one blame themselves. He just did not want to live and go on hurting. When he said this, his statement was punctuated by sobs, both his and his listeners. Tim reaffirmed his love for all.

For the first time, I shed my own long-dammed tears for my friend. The tape ended with Billy Joel again singing "Just the Way You Are".

The dark-skinned woman, Tim's sister, rose. A moistened handkerchief was her sole concession to grief as she told us that we could view the body.

Grace and I stood, joining the line that was headed by the mother of the fallen student-priest, a small thin woman, supported on either side by family members, sobbed. As she arrived at the coffin, she kissed her son's face continually. Only the gathered family stopped her from throwing herself violently upon her son's breast, as she called his name repeatedly. A gut-piercing wail rose from the woman's lips as she was led away protesting both the restraints of her family members and the immutability of death.

The line moved on slowly past the coffin of my stilled friend. Each person paused before Tim, some whispering farewells, others, like Grace, crying unabashedly. I did not stand long in front of the coffin. I had said my good-byes already.

At the door stood Tim's mother and sister, with other family members. The line of mourners passed before the family. Grace and I spoke briefly with Tim's roommate, Carl. I edged closer in the line, with Grace, toward Tim's mother. I searched my mind for something appropriate to say, something neither empty nor trite. In the seconds before we passed, her head bowed, caught in an outpouring of sorrow and tears. Of the languages and words I could have used, I realized that silence was the most eloquent. I said nothing.

□ □ □ □

I needed the solace, the calm, the refreshing vastness of the ocean. Though it was an hour out of our way, I used the coast route to return home.

Magenta ribbons spread across a turquoise sky as the setting sun fell headlong 0nto an azure sea.

CHAPTER 116

The only constant is Life. The dead come closest to remaining the same, but they too change with time in the minds of the living.
--a street-corner philosopher

Grace was leaving. I felt strangely impassive as I watched her load her belongings into our small yellow station wagon.

I helped very little. Though I had encouraged her leaving, I felt that packing and moving were her responsibility, this time. It was strange that once I had decided that the relationship would never work, the fighting, constant bickering had come to an abrupt end. We were more amicable living together in our non-relationship than we had ever been when we lived together as truly husband and wife.

The mental strain of seeing someone everyday about whom I had such ambivalent feelings was reaching the breaking point. Surges of resentment became increasingly more difficult to control. I felt put upon by Grace's presence, by my lack of privacy or freedom. I was beginning to feel good about myself again. My ties to Grace, filled with so many unpleasant remembrances, belonged to a time that I needed to leave behind.

I had called it fairness, my allowing her so many months to find a place of her own. Before that, I had called it economic necessity.

She took the last load out to the car. I leaned against the wall. I did not wish to sit. She returned. She took a last look around the apartment. She could find nothing that was hers there. With a saddened smile upon her face, she gave me a peck on the cheek. She turned to go.

The key, I reminded her. She took the small piece of metal off the ring. She placed it on the table. The high-pitched sound echoed oddly through the apartment.

When she had left, I sank into worn furniture, expecting a flood of the deepest depression to envelope me as it had before when Gracie left Instead, I felt a great relief. It was the last step in our physical separation and only the first in releasing her hold o my heart

CHAPTER 117

We are sorely needed and must find increasingly better ways to survive.

--a priest of the Semi-Secret Society of the Priests of the God of Life

The conference was an important one. Recruiters from all parts of the state were present. Part of the time was to be devoted to recruitment of pre-medical students for medical school. The remainder was to impart survival skills to newly-accepted student-priests entering medical school in the fall. Canon, whose performance on the National Board Examination had been legendary, had been asked to prepare a presentation on taking the exam.

The conference was important for other reasons, as well. Despite the near hysteria surrounding the Bakke case, the number of so called "minority" students in medical school was declining. Each medical school was pulling for a slice of a diminishing pie. The internal politics of Canon which had had the recruitment program on the brink of closing and which had produced state-wide lows in the number of entering freshmen had further worsened the problem. Canon was on the defensive. The other schools knew and took full advantage of this. Martha Livingston, director of the Office of

Minority Recruitment sent two of her best recruiters. Jack Franco, drove the university owned car as we arrived at the site of the conference. I had had only a passing acquaintance with the student priest. However, during the trials of the next several hours he earned my profound respect.

We were forced to give four successive forty-five minute talks as there was no room large enough to hold all the conference participants together. Midway during the second session our talk was sidetracked by medical students from neighboring schools who made several negative, misleading statements about Canon. Jack and I struggled for some time to counter these statements. After the session, one of the medical students who had given us a particularly hard time approached Jack and I. He grinned mischievously.

"You guys did pretty good up there."

"Yeah," I told him, "you sure didn't make it any easier for us." The three of us laughed.

□ □ □ □

A dinner and dance sponsored by the premedical society which had sponsored the conference was planned for the recruiters and newly-accepted student-priests.

I watched her dance. She liked to dance. Her step was light as she whirled around the dance floor. She was undoubtedly the prettiest and most interesting of the women present. Also, she was single. I reminded myself that I, too, was single again as my eyes followed her. I had never chosen to be involved with a woman whom I had found to be the most attractive in any setting. I had always allowed chance to make the choice. It was time I chose.

A life time of self perceived unattractiveness welled within me. My palms were suddenly moist as I searched for the courage with which to ask the woman for a dance. Nothing more, I told myself. After twenty nervous minutes, I asked her.

We danced and talked for some time. Soon we had exchanged numbers and had a date set for two weeks later when she would be visiting her brother who lived, as fate would have it, in Canon.

I smiled the entire trip back. I was healing. I was growing.

CHAPTER 118

"Why are we a secret society?"
"Because we allow our colleagues to ignore us."

--question of an initiate to the Semi-Secret Society of Priests of the God of Life.

I **was filled with** rage. Not again! A liberal string of expletives began as I read the signature at the bottom of the damning document which I had requested only as an afterthought. I read the first draft of a dean's letter which would make certain that not only would I be unable to find a residency, but that I would never practice medicine.

The dean's letter, a formal summary of the student's medical school career which often also contained the dean's opinion of the student was required by all residencies. It was a needed distillation of transcripts that were many times undecipherable. Since Canon was on a pass-fail system, and used no letter grades, the letter was of greater than usual importance.

I reread the maligning document again. The priest had taken particular care to selectively quote negative statements even when they lay in a sea of positive ones. Further he amplified on these statements until what was written had little relationship to the truth. I scanned the paper for some positive comments, for a favorable quote from a record which I knew had many. I found none.

More than the collective, prejudiced insult of the priest's summary of my medical school career was his last comment. It was one that no student who graduated from any medical school should have seen in their dean's letter.

He wrote, "In conclusion, . . . I cannot recommend this student to your program." It was a mean-spirited, petty, wholly unjustified act. The rancor, the contemptible nature of the priest's treachery fueled an anger which burned white-hot.

A few days later, I learned that Louis had been written an equally damning letter by another of the priests of Family Medicine.

When will it end? I thought.

□ □ □ □

I entered the Office of Student Affairs a step behind Garret Frank. I glared at the office staff as I entered, daring any to assume the smirks I had seen or imagined I had seen on too many similar occasions which had brought me to the office in the past.

Dr. Frank and I were there to see Richard Honeur, the new Associate Dean of Student Affairs. I knew the dean from the admissions committee which he had chaired. His easy charm, incisive intellect, and rapier sharp wit, along with what I had considered his conservative attitudes toward admissions had made him a formidable opponent. However, I had heard rumors about the new dean--all good. Students, particularly those of African and Hispanic descent, who presented legitimate complaints of mistreatment were finding rectification without resorting to the time-consuming procedure of faculty committees. I had not dealt with Honeur in his new capacity of dean, but the old distrust still remained.

I consoled myself with the knowledge that whatever else the dean was, he was also straightforward and honest. One knew exactly where one stood with the priest.

I expected a long, heated struggle to alter the contents of the letter written by the faculty member. That was alright. I was in a fit mood to manhandle a dean or anyone else. I also expected that he would have us wait to emphasize that he, the dean, was in control. I was surprised when we were shown directly into his office. I sank into a comfortable seat next to Garret Frank.

Perhaps sensing my barely controlled anger, the priest-confessor spoke first. He exchanged social amenities with the dean. I was strained, tense, fully prepared to take the dean's head off at the first errant word. Frank was calm, relaxed though he felt as strongly about the injustice of the letter as I. Involuntarily, a surge of admiration ran through me. Garret Frank knew how to handle himself. "Well, gentlemen, how can I help you." Honeur leaned back comfortably as he spoke. His tone was friendly, conversational.

"I think we need to discuss the nature and form of George's dean's letter." Frank spoke evenly.

The dean leaned forward. "I have to be honest with you, I haven't read the letter as yet." Though the dean's statement made sense, somehow it had not occurred to me that he had not read the letter. "Do you happen to have a copy of it with you?"

Frank handed my copy of the letter to Honeur. I could feel Franks mind working, waiting expectantly, as was mine, as we both watched the dean. Honeur's face clouded as he read the final sheet of the two-page document.

Dismay, anger, concern shone clearly on the high priest's face. He looked deep within my eyes. Ire rang in his voice. "This," he shook the paper, "would never have gone out over my signature." He handed the letter back to Frank.

The earnestness of the dean could not be denied.

The first document was discarded. An entirely new dean's letter was written.

Months later as I went on interviews and was told by several residency directors how strong my dean's letter was, I remembered the priest I had once counted as adversary and smiled.

CHAPTER 119

Life and Love are one. To serve either, we must remain faithful to both.
--from the Credo of the Society of
Semi-Secret Priests.

It was evening. The quiet in the large room was disturbed only by an occasional uniformed passer-by who sought some form of sustenance in the University Hospital cafeteria. Seeing the two freshly scrubbed faces of the student-priests in front of me brought back many memories. I had put off this meeting for some time. It was now overdue. I was both happy and sad.

The meeting for the election of officers had been called long in advance. The sparse attendance at the meeting belied the group's cohesiveness. The Canon chapter of the Student National Medical Association, the association of student-priests of African descent, was like most organizations. A small cadre performed the bulk of the work with the support of a much larger group. No one would dispute the election as those most interested in office were present. I did not envy the task ahead of the two students. It was an often time frustrating and lonely one.

The two student-priests, one born in mother Africa, the other in the strange land called America, watched me expectantly. I knew that look. I knew the things said and unsaid that they thought. I, not long before, had waited for the baton of power which I had felt, as they felt then, was my due.

This was the second time that I was president of the Canon chapter of the Student National Medical Association, the student arm of the Semi-Secret Society of Priests, was set to pass on the leadership of the organization to the student-priest who had served as vice-president. Tim's death, as it had been, he who had been slated to succeed me, had changed those plans. I had been left with no one to whom I might pass on the office.

It had been several months since I had called a meeting. My tenure as president had been fruitful, successful, but was clearly past its zenith. The medical school was no longer the focus of my life. I was looking forward to a residency and life away from the academy of Canon. The two student-priests knew this. I knew this. Still, I hesitated.

I spoke of mundane matters, went over a few sheets of the large cumbersome stack of papers of the Association.

Now, I know how Jimmy felt, I thought as I continued to delay. Jimmy had been president before me and had delayed interminably, it had seemed, before calling the election in which I had become president. Leadership of the organization was a responsibility which neither he nor I took lightly.

Neither of us wanted to see the spirit of the Twin Flames die.

I am only a link in a long chain, I reminded myself. I can but carry the burden which was mine and hope that those who came after me will carry theirs.

Already I had carried the burden a year beyond my time to allow these two student-priests to get beyond the pressure of the first year of medical school.

It was time that I move on. It was time that they assume their rightful positions of leadership.

I smiled at the two student-priests. I knew them well. As I sat before them, I thought, what is God except an ideal, a set of laws, honorable and inviolate, by which one lives?

I shared many values with all the priests of the House of Life. However, with the two who sat before me, I shared much more. I shared a profound and unshakable belief in a God whose spirit was embodied in the twin flames--Hope and Justice. The God of the Twin Flames was all the more important to me as I no longer believed in the God of the After-Life. For me, the God of the Twin Flames was the God of Life, the only God in which I could believe. The two before me had shown that they too believed in the God of the Twin Flames. As I handed the papers of the offices of the Semi-Secret Society to the two student-priests, I reached deep within the sheltered sacred alcove of my being where the Flames crackled over glowing embers. As I reached out, a flame in each hand, to the future priests who sat before me, fountains of fire burst forth from my two limbs. Three sets of brilliantly burning Flames appeared where before there had been one.

As I shook hands with the newly elected President and Vice-President, I realized that I would always be one of the Keepers of the Flame which grew ever brighter with giving.

CHAPTER 120

Upon completion of your training at the Academy, you are given the title doctor, or teacher. The knowledge and skills with which you go forth came not from within you, but were given freely by those who taught you as they were taught by those who passed before them.
You are not only empowered to teach, you are compelled to teach or the Priests of the God of Life will practice not healing arts, but dying arts.

--The Charging of the New Priests

A **hazy yellow sky** threatened sunshine. A familiar thought flashed briefly through my mind. Graduations, funerals, and weddings were events meant not for their chief participants, but for family and friends. I was concerned that an unhampered and unrelenting sun would be unleashed on my family before the ceremony ended. I worried most about my mother, who had recently developed high blood pressure. My family was present for my graduation from medical school. It was the culmination of one of their long-sought dreams.

Yes, it was their dream, too, I reminded myself as I turned to look at them. They sat in the first row of spectators. Love and pride shone brightly in eyes, focused not on the myriad of speakers, but on their own personal, soon to be graduated priest. The expressions of my family touched a part of me which had lain untouched for years. I smiled at them. The full, "smiling cheeks", as I called them, of my mother which were borne by each of her progeny as they returned my smile.

I heard their cheers and applause as I rose to receive my diploma. Soon after the reading of the Hippocratic oath, we retreated to the resplendently decorated cafeteria for the social portion of the gathering.

I was filled with a mixture of elation, sadness, and relief. I already missed my fellow students. I said many saddened good-byes. I drank long of faces, many of which I would never see again.

I reflected upon the many trials I had gone through and eventually overcome at the Academy of the Priests of the God of Life. I remembered how I had burned with thoughts of revenge against those who had tormented me. Yes, Frank was right. You know how far you have come when those who have hurt you were no longer important.

I had, my diploma, my first choice of residencies, the love of family and friends.

Already the trials were fading from memory. I had learned much during my travail in the priest academy. I had learned, largely from the priests, that there was no judgment as important as my own judgment of myself. I had learned that there was no pain that could not be overcome by hope, time, and the spirit of those human. I had learned that each of us is responsible for his own life and that the amount of suffering one bore was most often determined by the maltreatment to which one assents. I had learned that the joy of excelling far exceeded the meager half-fulfillment of passing. I had learned much at the academy. I had learned also that there was a time to go.

□ □ □ □

Eagle once-removed, fallen fawn, keeper of the tattered rainbow, these
Are my titles.

Sword-bearer, torch-holder, helper of humankind, lover of the earth, traveler. These, too, I am
called

Lover of the kind and giving,
lover of those who are loved and loving,
Believer in the tarnished gold of humanity, these also, am I.

Doctor, teacher of medicine, knight fallen from grace with himself,
knight of the broken armor,
blemished pride and unbroken courage. These, too, are
my titles.

Now behold, for despite all, it is time to forge yet another road. The time of parting has come. The long-sought dream is in hand.
Finally,

I am Priest.

THE THIRD YEAR

THE END

Cover art by Teresa Nieto

Made in the USA
Monee, IL
04 November 2026

67379936R00226